WHY PEOPLE GET SICK

AN EQUITY INITIATIVE PRODUCTION

WHY PEOPLE GET SICK

AND SOME MORE THAN OTHERS

**CLIVE TAN
PUTRI WIDI SARASWATI
EAINT THIRI THU**

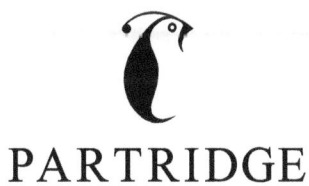

PARTRIDGE

Copyright © 2024 by Clive TAN
                    Putri Widi SARASWATI
                    Eaint Thiri THU.

Library of Congress Control Number: 2024902854
ISBN: Hardcover   978-1-5437-8250-9
              Softcover   978-1-5437-8089-5
              eBook   978-1-5437-8088-8

All rights reserved. No part of this book may be used or reproduced by any means, graphic, electronic, or mechanical, including photocopying, recording, taping or by any information storage retrieval system without the written permission of the author except in the case of brief quotations embodied in critical articles and reviews.

Because of the dynamic nature of the Internet, any web addresses or links contained in this book may have changed since publication and may no longer be valid. The views expressed in this work are solely those of the author and do not necessarily reflect the views of the publisher, and the publisher hereby disclaims any responsibility for them.

Print information available on the last page.

To order additional copies of this book, contact
Toll Free +65 3165 7531 (Singapore)
Toll Free +60 3 3099 4412 (Malaysia)
orders.singapore@partridgepublishing.com

www.partridgepublishing.com/singapore

Hear from our early readers

Why People Get Sick
And some more than others

Our well-being as humans is influenced by many factors, some of which we each can manage and influence, some of which may seem beyond our personal control. In clear, accessible and personal stories, "Why People Get Sick" illuminates these obstacles to the well-being of our communities and challenges and guides us to overcome them.

> - Mr Christopher G. Oechsli, President & CEO, Atlantic Philanthropies USA, Inc.

Through storytelling, the authors highlight how socio-economic factors, disasters, identity issues, and immigration challenges exacerbate health problems. Their poignant and heartfelt stories help readers to understand the inequities all around us and emphasize the need for fair health solutions to overcome systemic and financial barriers faced by marginalized communities.

> - Dr Le Nhan Phuong, Executive Director of The Equity Initiative Programme

"*The good physician treats the disease; the great physician treats the patient who has the disease.*" is a well-known aphorism attributed to Sir William Osler, described as the founder of modern medicine. In this wonderful collection of patient narratives, we are transported into the lives of our patients and people living with various health conditions, seeing life through their eyes. The reader appreciates the "*patient who has the disease*" and becomes a better clinician and human being. I hope this anthology is read by all who care for patients.

- Dr Jeremy Lim, Author of *Myth and Magic: The Singapore Healthcare System,* and President of the Precision Public Health Asia Society

All too often, medical education and health services focus solely on illnesses and ignore the social, economic and environmental factors that contribute to them. This book brings to life the complexities of health, and how the context where individuals come from and live in may significantly contribute to their health outcomes.

- Professor Dato' Dr Adeeba Kamarulzaman, President & Pro Vice-Chancellor, Monash University Malaysia

Social determinants of Health have been presented in many textbooks, but health workers at the grassroots level might not well understand its impact in real world settings. Through storytelling, this book shows how social determinant of health, especially the invisible and neglected ones, can devastate the health of individuals and community, and create health inequities at the population health level in Southeast Asia.
- Professor Chhea Chhorvann, Director of the National Institute of Public Health, Cambodia

This is a refreshingly honest and comprehensive take on the root causes of many ailments that plague modern day populations. The concept of equity is one that many governments and societies talk about, but seldom have concrete plans on achieving it. Health is what many people compromise when faced with difficult decisions in life.
- Professor Teo Yik Ying, Dean of Saw Swee Hock School of Public Health, National University of Singapore

Many areas of public policy are increasingly moving towards user- or citizen-centric approaches. In health and healthcare, this means keeping patients at the core of policies and programmes. This book is a shining example of the kind of rich, insightful and actionable knowledge that can emerge from such patient-centricity. The stories collected here are clear without being sentimental, rigorous without being rigid, and above all, wonderfully and informatively human.

- Dr Aaron Maniam, Fellow of Practice & Director, Digital Transformation Education, Blavatnik School of Government, University of Oxford, and Co-Chair, Global Future Council on Technology Policy, World Economic Forum

I am very excited to see this project come into fruition. This collection of powerful vignettes from individuals across Southeast Asia highlights the fact that social conditions determine health conditions. By sharing their stories, these resilient and courageous individuals challenge all of us to act in meaningful ways to address health inequity in our region.

- Associate Professor LE Minh Giang, Dean, School of Preventive Medicine and Public Health, Hanoi Medical University

CONTENTS

Introduction xi
Foreword xv

Story Of Amy | Citizenship 1
Story Of Habib | Displaced 8
Story Of Po Po Mok | Loneliness................. 15
Story Of Zhao (赵阿姨) | Deaf 21
Story Of Arun | Dementia............................29
Story Of Yap | Mental Wellbeing..................36
Story Of James | Magnetic 43
Story Of Afina | Epilepsy 50
Story Of Supap | Pollution 58
Story Of Rosa | Geography...........................65
Story Of Theresa | Conflict 72

About the Editors 79
About the Writers 81
Notes 85
Acknowledgements.................................... 107

INTRODUCTION

BY THE EDITORAL TEAM

Understanding why people get sick

So much of health is rooted in what is collectively known as social determinants of health. It means the conditions and environment in which people are born, grow, live, interact, work and age, and covers a wide range of factors such as socioeconomic status, education, employment, housing, residential status, migration history, sexuality, access to healthcare, social support networks, and even broader issues of conflict, disasters, poverty, colonization, and societal and cultural norms.

People with disadvantaged backgrounds often face barriers to good health. This means they get sick more easily, and it is harder for them to recover. A food delivery rider who had to work late nights is at higher risk of getting into a road traffic accident. Because of that, it impacts his/her ability to earn a good income, and they spiral further into poor physical and mental health.

Understanding health through an intersectional lens provides a more holistic understanding of why people get sick, and highlights the need for comprehensive and equitable solutions that address the complex realities of individuals and communities.

Talking about why people get sick

Being socially aware of these issues and disparities is the first step to talking about it and addressing these disparities to improve the health of our communities and sustainable health equity. If we agree that health is a basic human right, then we must work to build a world and society where everyone has a fair and equitable opportunity to attain their highest level of health.

We cannot assume that people know about these issues, or know how to talk about these issues. We believe it is important to start somewhere. Not with theories, but with stories. Stories that are real, stories that are relatable, stories that are from Asia, by Asia. These stories are by young people, for young people, and the young at heart. We hope that for you the reader, each story will be a discovery, as they illustrate how health inequities are shaped by a multitude of intersecting factors, including identity, socioeconomic status, employment, social isolation, and family dynamics, which individually and collectively create barriers to accessing quality healthcare and contribute to poorer health outcomes.

We hope that these stories will move you, as there is no motion without emotion, give you more understanding of the context, and provide you with the momentum, language and initiative to talk confidently with others about these issues. And if your friend or colleague is wondering why people get sick, you can share your knowledge and this book with them, for "a candle loses nothing by lighting another candle". Let's spread the word, build collective empathy, and together let us build towards a brighter future for tomorrow.

Clive TAN
Putri Widi SARASWATI
Eaint Thiri THU

FOREWORD

BY DR ROGER GLASS
AND DR BARBARA STOLLS

Most countries, both rich and poor, experienced a nearly doubling of the life expectancy of their populations from 30-45 years in 1900 to 60-80 years by the year 2022. A century of improvements in knowledge about diseases, their spread, prevention and cure led to these improvements. Coupled with advances in programs for sanitation and health, education (particularly for women), economic development and more, this expanded knowledge base catalyzed an era of transformative advances in the prevention and treatment of major illnesses.

Throughout the world, the impact of these remarkable advances has not been shared equally. Differences in economic and social status, urban versus rural residence, ethnicity, education level, and other factors leave many groups behind. Taking action to increase health equity – making quality healthcare accessible to all – can be a daunting and sometimes uncomfortable challenge. It asks us to explore the underlying reasons why the promise of healthier lives remains stubbornly out of reach for some groups and beckons us to commit resources to develop and implement novel interventions to bring down barriers. Greater focus on the social determinants of health and disease —the non-medical factors that influence health outcomes – is essential. One way is to draw on the power of storytelling, using an individual's story to shed light on broader issues.

This collection of short vignettes from a variety of settings in Southeast Asia provides personal insights into why people get sick and the physical and emotional toll of health inequities. These stories were brought together by three senior fellows of the Equity Initiative, a program launched by CMB in 2016 to enhance the leadership skills of a diverse group of professionals working within their own communities to promote heath equity and social justice. In bringing this book to life, Clive Tan (Singapore), Putri Widi Saraswati (Indonesia), and Eanit Thiri Thu (Myanmar) remind us of the challenges that must be addressed to fulfill the promise of better health for all.

Roger I. Glass, M.D., Ph.D.
President, CMB

AND

Dr Barbara Stolls, M.D., PhD
    Immediate Past President, CMB

Why People Get Sick

AND SOME MORE THAN OTHERS

STORY OF AMY

CITIZENSHIP

"My leg is really painful but there's no way I can take another day off from work again." I said to myself as I limped to take the bus to the childcare centre. I worked as a childcare attendant in my son's childcare centre. This is the first job I ever have in Singapore. My son's principal is very kind to offer this job to me when I mentioned to her that it is really difficult for a foreigner like me to find work.

However, it has not been easy. I struggled in the job as I am not able to stand long with my painful knees. I also have frequent headaches which is making me not able to focus on my job. The frequency of headaches is now almost on a daily basis. I am worried as I don't know what is happening to me. I went to the nearby family doctor and he had given me some painkillers and a letter to see the hospital specialist. The painkillers now no longer work as my pain is getting more intense. I wanted to go to the hospital specialist but my husband said "next month" as this month we need to pay for my elder boy's new school uniform. However, last month he also told me the same thing that he needs to spend his salary on some other expenses.

Many times, I asked myself whether I have made the right decision to marry my husband. I am from Indonesia. After my first husband passed away, my son was only 5 years old then. Though life was difficult, I could still make a living by selling some food on the streets. I met my current husband through some friends. He is a Singaporean and told me he has a stable job in Singapore and will be able to take good care of me and my son. Furthermore, he told me that my son will have a brighter future if he can go to school in Singapore. It's scary to uproot myself from Indonesia since this is where my friends and family are. If I go to Singapore, I don't know anyone and I can't even speak a word of proper English. However, the moment I think that my son can have a brighter future in Singapore, I accepted my husband's proposal and followed him to Singapore.

Initially, my husband was very nice to me and my son. He treated my son as his own son. He does not earn a high pay as a security guard but he tried his best to pay for his expensive school fees since he is an Indonesian and not eligible for any subsidies for his school fees. We then had another son and he was born deaf. Luckily, this son is a Singaporean and is entitled to subsidies and financial aid. If not, I don't think we will be able to afford his hearing aid, his therapist fees and special school fees.

However, my life crumbled bit by bit when my husband got retrenched and was not able to get a proper job. We are stressed and we always quarrel over money. He always blames that my first son's school fees are too expensive. I tried my best to apply for financial help for his school fees but all the social workers will always tell me that they can't do much since he's a foreigner. The social workers tried to help us to apply for permanent residency for my son and myself twice in Singapore, however they have not been successful and the application fees are also expensive.

I then think of ways of how I can earn more money. I am a good cook so I started to cook delicious Indonesian food at home and sell it online. However, the money I earned from the cooking is not significant as I am not able to cope with big orders since I don't even have the capital to buy the ingredients first. Furthermore, I am not able to stand long to do the cooking due to my painful swollen legs. Therefore, I am thankful that I am able to get the childcare attendant job even though I can't even converse very well in English. However, I am really not sure how long I can hold on to the job. Every day I struggled with leg pain and headache. I know I need to go to the specialist to get proper treatment but there's no way we can afford the fees. I don't want to borrow any more money from people as we already have lots of debts. I am a foreigner and I am tired of hearing social workers telling me that they can't help to apply for any subsidies or assistance.

People ask me to go back to Indonesia but it's even worse back there. I also need to go to a private hospital in Indonesia to get proper treatment and the fees are also not cheap. I also cannot leave my sons in Singapore without anyone to care for them. I don't think I can trust my husband to take good care of them.

I just pray that nothing serious is happening to me and hopefully they will all go away.

Story by Lena

What happened in the Story of Amy?

Amy is dealing with persistent leg pain and frequent headaches, which are affecting her ability to work. She has been prescribed painkillers, but they are no longer effective, and she needs to see a hospital specialist. However, financial constraints are preventing her from seeking further treatment. For Amy, her relationship with her current husband is also strained due to financial stress and their son's medical needs. Her job as a childcare attendant is physically demanding, and her limited English skills make it even more challenging. Despite the numerous challenges, Amy displays resilience and determination. She tries various ways to earn money, such as selling Indonesian food online, to support her family. Her commitment to her children's well-being and their future is evident, even as she grapples with her own health issues.

This story reflects the challenges many foreigners face in finding employment and accessing affordable healthcare in a new country. Healthcare costs are heavily subsidised by the government in many countries. This helps to keep the cost of healthcare services low for its citizens and is aligned with the push by the World Health Organisation for universal health coverage (UHC). Even as the cost of healthcare services continue to rise with inflation and more advanced technology and treatments, governments have been able to keep up with the level of subsidies and keep healthcare costs affordable for most of its citizens.

However foreign spouses with children that do not have citizenship are in a vulnerable position. This is not unique to Singapore, but in Singapore the price difference between subsidised healthcare and non-subsidised healthcare in the public healthcare sector can be very significant. Foreign spouses of low-income citizens have reduced access to job opportunities, and face financial barriers when it comes to accessing healthcare services.

Low-cost preventive health services and routine basic medical services that are accessible to citizens are not subsidised for these foreign spouses, and they become costly and inaccessible. Even when they get sick, many withhold or avoid a visit to the general practitioner or specialist because of the high costs involved. Often their health worsens due to the lack of timely medical attention and they do not recover from their sickness. By the time they see the doctor, they are often severely ill.

Thinking about why people get sick

Many foreign spouses and children in low-income households suffer from similar situations. They are in "no man's land" as they are not a citizen in the country they reside in, but going back to their home country for medical review and treatment is also not a viable solution. Understanding the intersection of identity (e.g. gender, race, immigration status) and health, do we see how these factors and structural barriers can impact an individual's access to healthcare and overall well-being?

Given the importance of social connections and community support in maintaining good health, how did the family dynamics and the lack of a support system affect Amy's health and well-being?

Who are the stakeholders in one's country and society that can contribute to making a difference to these vulnerable and marginalised people?

Ten years from now – what would be the future that we can imagine for this group of foreign spouses and children in low-income households in your country? How would the situation be different?

Given the settings and the financial constraints, if you were in her position, how would you prioritize your health needs?

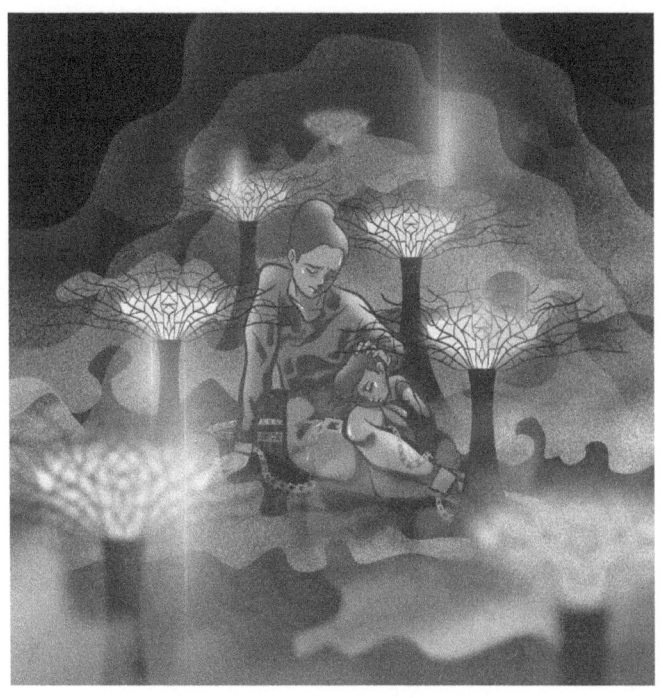

Illustrated by Jelita Alima Rembulan
LinkedIn: linkedin.com/diasijelita \ linktr.ee/diasijelita

STORY OF HABIB

DISPLACED

At the age of 26, I was leading a tranquil life in my village. All that tranquility was swept away by the eruption of a brutal conflict, forcing me to abandon the land I loved so dearly. With a heart filled with fear and uncertainty, I started a perilous journey with my family, heading for Bangladesh in hope of refuge.

Under the concealment of the night, my wife, our newborn child, and I navigated the forests and difficult terrains. Our migration journey was filled with the chilling echoes of gunfire and heart-wrenching cries of those left behind. The journey was difficult with numerous hurdles and terror-filled moments, with each step a gamble of life as we made our way towards the refuge of the border. Completely drained and mentally distressed, we eventually set foot in Bangladesh, our sanctuary.

In the refugee camp, I found myself rebuilding my life from nothing. My health waned as I scavenged for materials to build a shelter for my family, and every day was a battle. With resources scarce, my determination and the support of my Rohingya brothers were the only things that helped us create a sense of normalcy in the camp.

Over time, our situation started to improve, if only slightly. Aid groups and humanitarian organizations took notice of our dire conditions and offered their assistance. The construction of sanitary latrines and the delivery of aid provided us with a faint glimmer of hope. However, our mobility was always restricted, trapping us in a cycle of uncertainty within the camp.

My child almost died in the camp. Doctors told us that he had contracted a coughing disease (Diphtheria). Many children got the disease at the same time, and everyone was worried. By the grace of Allah, he survived. In November 2021, I also suddenly became severely ill and could not even walk properly. After lying in bed for almost 1 week, I finally managed to gather the courage to see a doctor who told me that I was suffering from Dengue. I was provided with some medications and recovered after struggling for several weeks with fatigue and body ache. Such is our life in the camp, because so many of us live in the same area, when there is a disease, many people get sick.

The year 2023 brought with it a fresh calamity. News of reduced aid reached our camp and spread like wildfire. The international agencies' decision to cut our monthly food allocation further aggravated our already desperate situation, pushing us to the brink of starvation. The women and children in our camp, including my family, would suffer the most as a result of this decision.

Torn between my love for my family and the need to provide for them, I considered the risky journey on an illegal boat to Malaysia for work. With dwindling international aid, local people in Bangladesh became increasingly hostile to us, adding to our misery. Our resilience as Rohingyas was put to the test every day as we struggle with starvation and the harsh reality of living as outsiders. There are no jobs for us, violence is a daily occurrence and incidents of arson in the camps were not uncommon.

Humanitarian agencies say that they are pleading for support, appealing for the necessary funds to assist us Rohingya refugees. They tell us that they are telling the world of our urgent need for international intervention, arguing that countless lives, including mine, were hanging in the balance. Despite their efforts, however, they say that funds remain insufficient. We are left in a state of extreme vulnerability.

*Note: This narrative is intended to shed light on the challenging circumstances faced by Rohingya refugees and the necessity for ongoing humanitarian assistance. It encapsulates their resilience amidst adversity and underscores the importance of global solidarity and support to mitigate their hardship.

Story by Collins SANTHANASAMY

What happened in the Story of Habib?

Habib's story begins with him being forced to flee his village due to conflict, reflecting the tragic reality of many Rohingya refugees. The description of his journey to Bangladesh is filled with fear, uncertainty, and life-threatening challenges. Navigating through forests and difficult terrain, under the cover of night, highlights the dangerous nature of their migration. The echoes of gunfire and cries of those left behind paint a harrowing picture of the violence and trauma they experienced.

Upon reaching Bangladesh, Habib finds himself starting anew in a refugee camp. The initial focus is on survival and creating a sense of normalcy. Habib's health suffers as he scavenges for materials to build a shelter for his family, showcasing the physical toll of displacement. Over time, aid groups and humanitarian organizations provide some relief by constructing sanitary latrines and delivering aid. However, the camp still faces challenges, including the outbreak of diseases like Diphtheria, which almost took the life of Habib's child. The spread of such diseases in crowded and unsanitary living conditions is a common issue in refugee camps. Additionally, Habib's personal battle with Dengue fever underscores the vulnerability of refugees to infectious diseases.

Conflict and disasters caused by natural, man-made and technological hazards often cause displacement of populations – sometimes temporary, sometimes for much longer than what is bearable. Internally displaced persons (IDPs) and refugees caught in the crossfire of these human conflicts, suffer not only the loss of their homes and livelihoods but also endure the dire consequences of poor health that accompany their displacement.

Refugees and internally displaced persons often have to reside in overcrowded makeshift camps or are forced to seek shelter in abandoned buildings. In these cramped conditions, diseases can spread easily. Limited healthcare infrastructure and accessibility contribute to health inequities, as refugees may not receive timely or specialized care, leading to poorer health outcomes.

Basic necessities become luxuries, and access to clean water, food, and healthcare becomes a daily struggle. Within the camps they face restricted mobility and uncertainty, they are unable to freely move or seek better opportunities. This sense of confinement adds to the mental distress and uncertainty about their future. Their mental health is further exacerbated by experiencing the trauma of conflict and loss of their loved ones. The ripple effects of conflict, displacement, and inadequate resources all converge to cause deterioration of health for these persons and their families.

Habib's story serves as a powerful reminder of the resilience and strength displayed by refugees in the face of tremendous challenges. It highlights the complex interplay of factors affecting their lives, including conflict, displacement, healthcare, sanitation, and limited resources. His story is a call for continued attention and support to mitigate the hardships endured by people displaced by conflict.

Thinking about why people get sick

Habib's identity as a Rohingya refugee is central to his story and intersects with his health and well-being. When refugees flee their homeland and seek refuge in neighboring countries, their lives and communities are disrupted, and they often face poverty, unemployment, and limited access to education, healthcare and social services.

How can we better acknowledge the devastating consequences of human conflict and the toll it takes on the health of refugees and internally displaced persons? What are some things that our local community can do to show our support for these internally displaced persons – even though they may be many miles away?

Closer to home – are there people in our community or neighbourhood who are "displaced" for a different set of reasons, and are they suffering from negative health effects due to their "displaced" status?

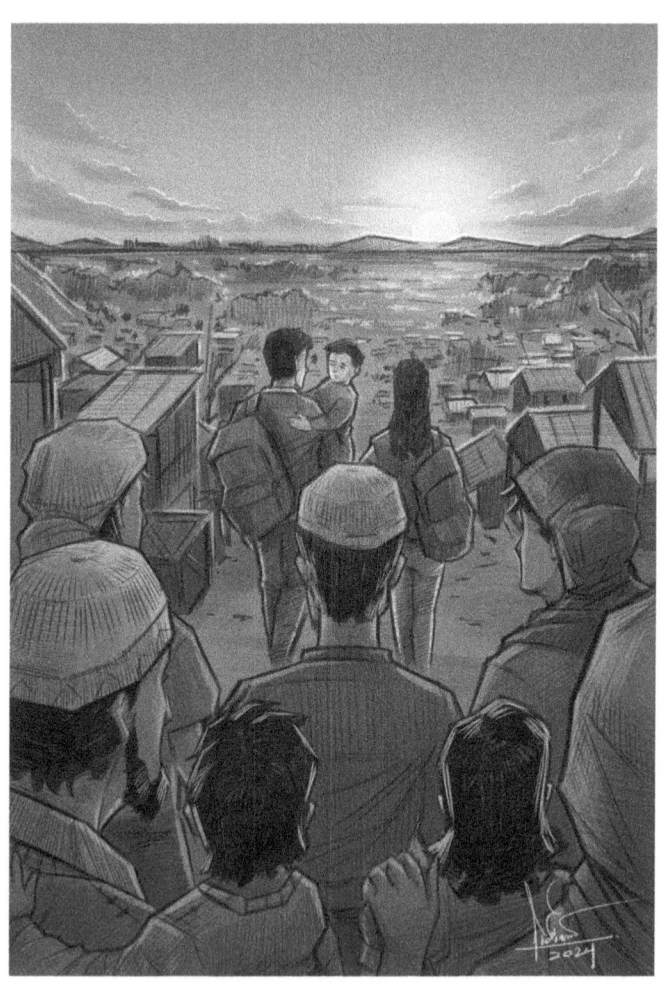

Illustrated by Ye Min Htet

STORY OF PO PO MOK

LONELINESS

It is one of those evenings. I find myself, once again, sitting at the cool stone bench outside my apartment. I don't like to join the chats with my neighbours; I prefer to sit by myself. Occasionally when my younger friends visit (I don't have that many younger friends), and when I am in a mood to talk, I sometimes lament to them that, "When a person grows older there is really nothing much to look forward to; I'm just waiting to die."

I feel helpless and hopeless. One night my younger friend asked me why I kept thinking about death and dying. I reflected deeply and decided to share with her my life story. Ever since my son passed away, I can't stop thinking about him, about how we used to care for one another. I feel very lonely now that he is no longer around. I miss him very much and I often wonder why such an unfortunate thing had happened to me. My younger friend listened attentively and said nothing and she reached out to hold my hand in hers. I felt comforted, for the first time in many months – I was able to share my grieve with another human that genuinely cared. This season of bereavement is like walking through a dark forest, not knowing when and if I will ever get out of it. I don't have much appetite these days and I often wish that my days on earth will end soon. Even though I had food delivered to my doorstep by one of those organisations, the box of "菜販" (vegetables and rice) tasted bland; I would rather sleep than eat alone. I eat simply, usually some biscuits and milo; these are enough to fill my stomach.

Another one of those evenings where I had the occasional visitor. My younger friends helped me to boil water and refilled the water flask so that I can use at night. I smiled and said good night. I was lying in bed that night and thinking why they would show kindness to me? I feel unseen and unheard most of my days. Nobody is interested in talking with me; aging alone is lonely and painful. My daughter who has relocated to Canada doesn't want me, my husband and son has passed on before me. What is there to look forward to each day? Will I wake up again to another day of loneliness? Another day of pain? Will there be any light at the end of the tunnel? How will I live going forward? I don't feel connected with my neighbours, I don't feel that there is a reason to live.

Story by Jun

What happened in the Story of Mok?

Mok's advanced age intersects with her experience of profound grief, creating a unique set of challenges. Older adults often face increased vulnerability to physical and mental health issues. The loss of her son, husband, and the distance from her daughter have left Mok feeling lonely and hopeless. The lack of social connections and feelings of disconnection from her neighbors contribute to Mok's loneliness. Mok's sense of isolation and loneliness are key factors influencing both her physical and mental health.

Both loneliness and social isolation, especially in older adults, are associated with increased mortality (higher risk of death), increased risk of depression, cognitive decline and physical health issues, and poorer health outcomes. Although they are not the same thing, they are both common among older adults, and have severe health and social consequences. Studies have shown that risk of an earlier death from a lack of social connection is greater than that from obesity.

Older adults who do not have trusted family members or friends whom they can share their burdens with, in times of need may be at higher risk of loneliness, social isolation, depressive symptoms and poor health outcomes. Limited social support, especially for older adults, can exacerbate feelings of loneliness and depression. Social connections and supportive relationships are crucial for maintaining mental and physical health. In Mok's situation, she feels unseen and unheard by her neighbors, indicating a lack of social connectedness. However, the support and kindness shown by her younger friends bring her comfort.

The loss of loved ones and the sense of loneliness have left Mok struggling to find purpose and meaning in her daily life. Purpose and meaning are important components of overall well-being. The absence of meaningful activities and connections can contribute to a decline in mental and physical health, as individuals may lose their sense of identity and motivation.

Thinking about why people get sick

Mok's story provides insight into the complex interplay between aging, grief, loneliness, and their impact on health. By understanding the intersectional factors contributing to poorer health outcomes, people can work towards creating more supportive and equitable environments for older persons in our communities.

Mok's story underscores the health inequities faced by older adults, particularly those experiencing grief and isolation, and highlights the potential gap in mental health services for older adults. Older adults may face barriers to accessing mental healthcare, including stigma, lack of awareness, and limited mobility. The intersection of aging and mental health underscores the need for tailored mental health services and support systems for this vulnerable population. Are you aware of any potential barriers older adults may face in accessing mental healthcare services in your community?

How does the experience of profound grief, like the loss of a loved one which is common in the elderly, impact one's mental health? Are there any vulnerable elderly or other groups in your community who are at risk of social isolation and loneliness? Are there any local statistics or monitoring of this issue?

For example, a Singapore Ministry of Health report in 2021 shared that there were 400 cases of suicide in 2019, of which 122 cases involved persons 60 years and above.

How can we work together with communities and public service agencies do better to identify and reduce the prevalence of loneliness and social isolation in these vulnerable groups of elderly in our communities?

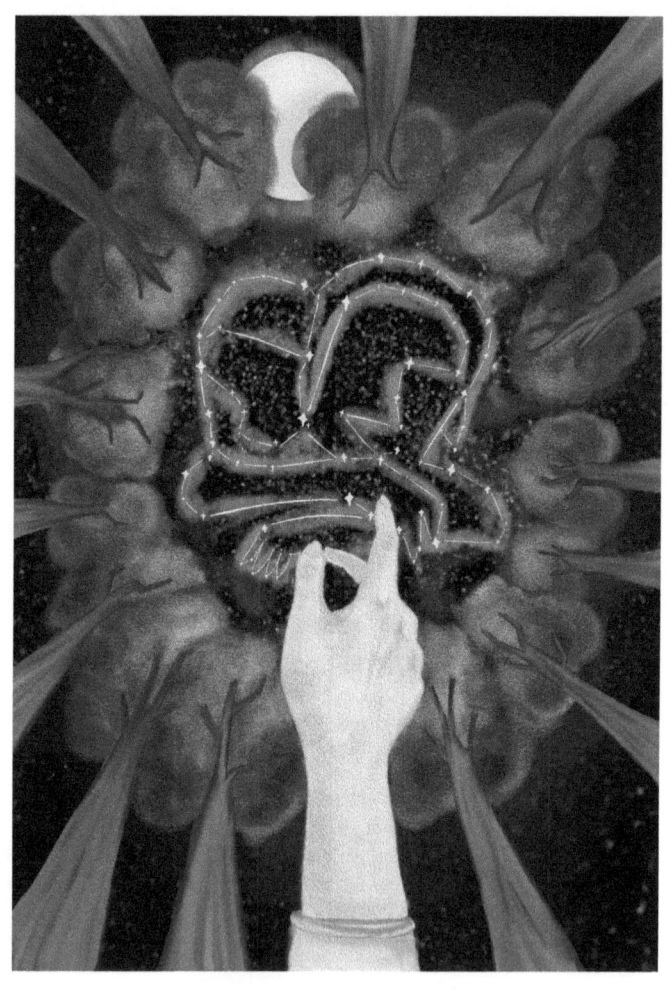

Illustrated by Norena Darsana
LinkedIn: linkedin.com/norena-darsana-885052164
Instagram: @northetutor

STORY OF ZHAO（赵阿姨）

DEAF

I am 62 years old, and had been married to my husband for 40 years. Both of us are deaf. I have a daughter, who has normal hearing.

My belly had not been feeling well in the last three years but I hate to go hospital where punishment is waiting. Here is why:

In the summer of 2019, there is one time that I felt much pain in my belly. I felt very bad and ask my daughter what to do. She does not know sign language, just a bit of the basics. She said I could go with her for a health check. But she does not stay with me and works in another side of Beijing. I had to wait for another three days for her to come accompany me to see the doctor at the hospital. She helped me to do the registration online in advance and we waited for two hours just for our term. The consultation process only took 10 minutes. I wondered whether it worth the money we have paid. During the consultation, I described my pain with my unclear pronunciation. I want him to know that I had diarrhoea, and my back also hurt badly in recently months. I want him to know that the pain in my belly was so bad that I could not eat well and was terribly upset. I want to tell the doctor the whole story and my health situation.

What annoyed me was that the doctor only talked to my daughter. I think he could not understand my pronunciation. She tried very hard to help explain what I was saying to him. We waited for two hours while the doctor only gave us 10 minutes. His indifferent and impatient expression says it all. We left with some painkillers. My daughter and I felt very disappointed and humiliated by the healthcare team.

After only a month, I felt that I should see the doctor again. The painkillers did not work. I did not want to bother my daughter again and just went to the hospital with my husband. When we arrived, the nurses on the front desk said we needed to do medical registration in advance. I saw that there were many doctors around, and begged the nurses to send someone to treat me as I was in pain. They replied that the doctors were busy and asked my husband to help fill up the registration form. It was such a difficult conversation for both of us as we are deaf, and no one in the hospital could understand sign language. We tried to plead with them for their help, but finally we gave up and returned home sadly.

I learnt that I need to bring in some who could write. In the previous episode, I recalled that my daughter helped me to do medical registration two days in advance. Again, I did not want to bother my daughter, so I asked my nephew to come with me. He is also deaf, but he can read and write. We went to the hospital on time, and finally met with the same doctor who treated me last time. He told us in writing that we should have a complete X-ray examination and blood test. I was very worried when I heard that. I did not trust the doctor's plan to do these additional tests. I was worried that it would be too complicated to find where to go in the big hospital, and it would take me hours to just do one check. Besides I doubt whether the doctor really understood what I was talking about and what was causing my pain.

What happened next was a disaster for the two of us. We moved around from one building to another, paid for the bills in one place, and then went for the blood tests in another place. We do not recognize the hospital signs (we cannot read) and the different nurses gave us complicated instructions and directions (we are deaf) which made it very confusing. We took three hours to move around many places in the hospitals, it was stressful, frustrating, and exhausting. Finally, we gave up on doing the test and examination.

In the last three years I still have much pain in my belly, but I do not want to go back to the hospital again. I will eat some biscuits and sometime just drink hot water to calm it down.

Luckily, I found a sign language interpreter this March and she helped me to navigate through the hospital processes to see the doctor. The result was that I got a tumor in my uterus and had serious gastritis. The doctor explained the situation was not good and commented that it would not have gotten so bad if I had done my test and examination on time and received the treatment earlier.

I was shocked, angry and humiliated, and wished that I had met the sign language interpreter earlier.

Story by ZHOU Haibin

What happened in the Story of Zhao?

Zhao's story sheds light on the unique challenges faced by individuals with disabilities when accessing healthcare services. Zhao, who is deaf, encounters significant communication barriers when seeking medical attention. The inability of healthcare providers to understand her sign language creates a major obstacle to effective communication. Her experience highlights the lack of accessibility and special arrangements for individuals with hearing impairments in healthcare settings. This can lead to frustration, miscommunication, misunderstanding, and potential misdiagnosis.

Many patients with hearing disabilities like Zhao may often feel that they do not understand the medical system and processes. They want to tell the doctor all their symptoms and problems in one sitting and hope that one doctor can cure all their sicknesses. When the doctor does a referral, they can often misunderstand the process and have the perception that the doctor is discriminative and wishes to avoid treating deaf patients.

When the deaf patient is in the clinic or ward, the doctors and nurses would feel that it is easier to talk to the patients' relatives who can speak, such as Zhao's daughter or the sign language interpreter. Often they would simply hear part of the story from the relatives or interpreter, and miss out on double-checking with the patient themselves. In between, much information on what was important for the patients would be lost in translation. To make things worse, the patients' anxieties often bubble up when they do not feel heard.

In this situation, we can see that Zhao's hearing disability directly impacts her access to healthcare. The absence of sign language interpreters or staff proficient in sign language creates barriers to effective communication and understanding of medical instructions. The complexity of hospital procedures and the need for multiple tests further exacerbates the challenges for individuals with hearing disabilities.

Persons with hearing disabilities may often delay their treatment when the medical services are not accessible. Not many hospitals have staff who are trained in sign language. The many barriers in place mean that many persons with hearing disabilities like Zhao would delay seeking medical advice for their symptoms. Due to the communication barriers and navigation challenges, Zhao's health condition worsened over three years. Her initial symptoms of abdominal pain and diarrhea were not adequately addressed, leading to late presentation of the illness when it becomes very serious and difficult to neglect. The delay in diagnosis and treatment resulted in her tumor and gastritis becoming more severe. In the case of Zhao, she lost three years' of opportunity to get her sickness treated in a timely manner. This highlights the potential consequences of inaccessible healthcare for individuals with disabilities.

Thinking about why people get sick

Zhao's experience highlights the intersection of disability and healthcare access. How do communication barriers impact the health outcomes of individuals with disabilities?

As a deaf individual, Zhao encounters significant communication barriers when seeking medical attention. The lack of sign language interpretation and accessible communication methods creates a major obstacle to understanding her health condition and navigating the healthcare system. It is useful to reflect and ask ourselves if our community and society is sensitive to the health needs and accessibility of our medical services for people with hearing disabilities?

The process of medical registration and navigating the hospital premises presents significant challenges for Zhao and her husband who also has hearing impairment. What are some of the good practices that our community have put in place to be more sensitive to the health needs of the hearing impaired community? How can our healthcare providers exercise empathy and patience toward their patients with hearing disabilities?

Understanding of the unique challenges faced by individuals with disabilities in the healthcare system and the importance of accessible communication, advocacy, and person-centered care, who are the people or groups in our community who are concerned about, advocating for and speaking up for the people living with such disabilities, and emphasizing on the importance of disability-inclusive healthcare services? Why is it important to have someone or an organization to advocate for this group?

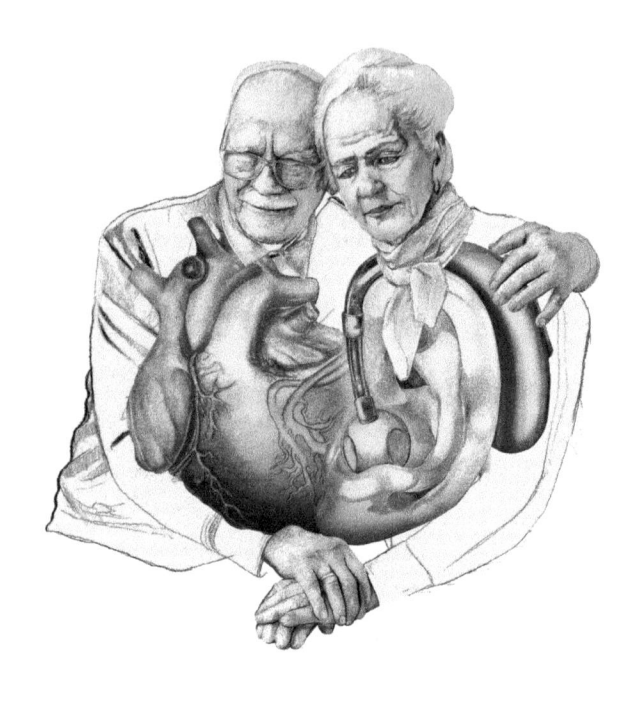

Illustrated by Anzi Matta
Instagram: @anzimatta | anzimatta.com

STORY OF ARUN

DEMENTIA

"Alzheimer's disease." The doctor stated the diagnosis for my mother. She was 70 years old. I was 42 years old; this was the first time I heard of the condition, but it all made sense. She asked me everyday to buy her a new phone. I bought one for her already but she forgot how to use it so she thought it was broken. She was becoming more forgetful. We did not know what to do, how to help my mother get better. We lived in a suburb area near Bangkok. My family and neighbours did not know how to help or treat people with Alzheimer's, and we did not know who to ask. Her condition gradually worsened.

One day she went out to the store by herself and got lost. We were so worried. After many hours of searching, my sister and I found her wandering around at the mall and brought her back home. After that, the house door had to always be locked with the key. We did not want to lock her at home, but we had to work and could not stay at home with her the whole day. Yes we were worried, but we were more worried that she might get lost again. It did not seem like the right thing to do, but we did not know of a better way. We felt alone and isolated.

Before all this happened, our family factory went out of business and we had to sell our house and move into a much smaller house further away from the city. With the new mortgage payments for the house, we were barely making ends meet and there was no money for me to bring my mother to see the specialist.

When the year of Covid-19 pandemic arrived. I lost my job and hustled. Luckily a few months later I could get a delivery job when the town started to open up. That helped my family get through the tough situation a lot.

But things can always get worse. My father was diagnosed with liver cancer. We took him to the emergency room the day his eyes were looking up at the ceiling and not responding. My mother's condition also got worse. She started not to remember how to eat, use the bathroom, talk in sentences, and many more things. I wish there was something we could do to help my mother get better. My sister and I also had less time and resources to take care of our mother. We had to work hard to earn money, while trying to save more money to help our father survive his cancer.

Story by Katie Kanyarat FERGUSON

What happened in the Story of Arun?

Arun's story highlights the intersection of Alzheimer's disease, a progressive brain disorder, and the caregiving challenges faced by families. Alzheimer's impacts not only the individual with the diagnosis but also their caregivers, in this case, Arun and his sister. The physical and mental demands of caring for a loved one with a progressive disease create a unique set of health inequities and challenges.

Arun and his sister juggle caregiving responsibilities while also needing to work, reflecting the intersection of caregiving and employment. Caregivers often experience role strain, where the demands of caregiving conflict with their work responsibilities. The emotional toll of caring for loved ones with Alzheimer's and cancer is evident in Arun's story. Caregiver strain can lead to reduced work productivity, financial strain, and increased stress, impacting their physical and mental health.

The family's decision to restrict Arun's mother's freedom by locking the house door showcases the complex balance between safety and autonomy. Caregivers may need to implement restrictive measures to ensure the safety of their loved ones, but these measures can also impact the mental health and well-being of both the caregivers and the individual with Alzheimer's.

The financial situation of Arun's family contributes to health inequities. Financial constraints can force individuals to prioritize work over their well-being, often resulting in the neglect of their health and a negative spiral of declining physical and mental well-being. For Arun, the loss of their family business and subsequent financial struggles limited their ability to access specialized healthcare for both Arun's mother and father. Financial barriers can lead to delayed treatment, inadequate care, and increased stress for caregivers, potentially impacting their overall health and well-being.

The progressive nature of Alzheimer's disease underscores the need for specialized care and interventions. As the disease worsens, individuals may require memory clinics, dementia care specialists, or residential care settings. Access to these specialized services can be limited or financially challenging. Families facing Alzheimer's often require guidance, resources, and emotional support. The lack of knowledge about Alzheimer's disease in Arun's community highlights health inequities related to education and support systems, and underscore the need for community education and accessible support services for caregivers.

Many Thai individuals continue to rely heavily on their faith. They perceive unfavorable circumstances as signs of bad luck and mistakenly believe that social assistance is scarce, leading them to adopt a defeatist attitude towards sickness and health. Some people have suggested that there is a perceived lack of organized efforts to provide support and raise awareness among those who require assistance. Consequently, there are needy individuals who are left to either seek help independently or erroneously assume that no aid is available to them. In Thailand, there are organizations such as Alzheimer's Association but Arun was not aware of them, explaining that neither the doctor nor the nurses at the hospital shared this information with him.

Thinking about why people get sick

Arun's experience highlights the intersection of how caring for a family member with gradually worsening Alzheimer's Disease while being financially constrainted can lead to high caregiver strain and burden, and negatively impact the physical and mental health of the caregivers. Through Arun's story, we can gain a deeper understanding of the complex dynamics between caregiving, healthcare access, community support, and the potential consequences of health inequities on individuals and their caregivers.

In our community, do we observe situations where caregiving responsibilities had negatively impact the health and well-being of caregivers? What do we see as the potential long-term effects of caregiving responsibilities on caregivers' mental and physical health, especially when coupled with financial constraints? How do communication barriers impact the health outcomes of individuals with disabilities?

In our community and city, are we able to find community resources for people living with Alzheimer's

Disease in your community? Why is community education and support crucial for families facing Alzheimer's disease?

In our community, are there specialized care for people with progressive diseases like Alzheimer's? Are these services accessible to people who need them – both geographically and financially? What potential barriers can we identify for persons or family members who need these services?

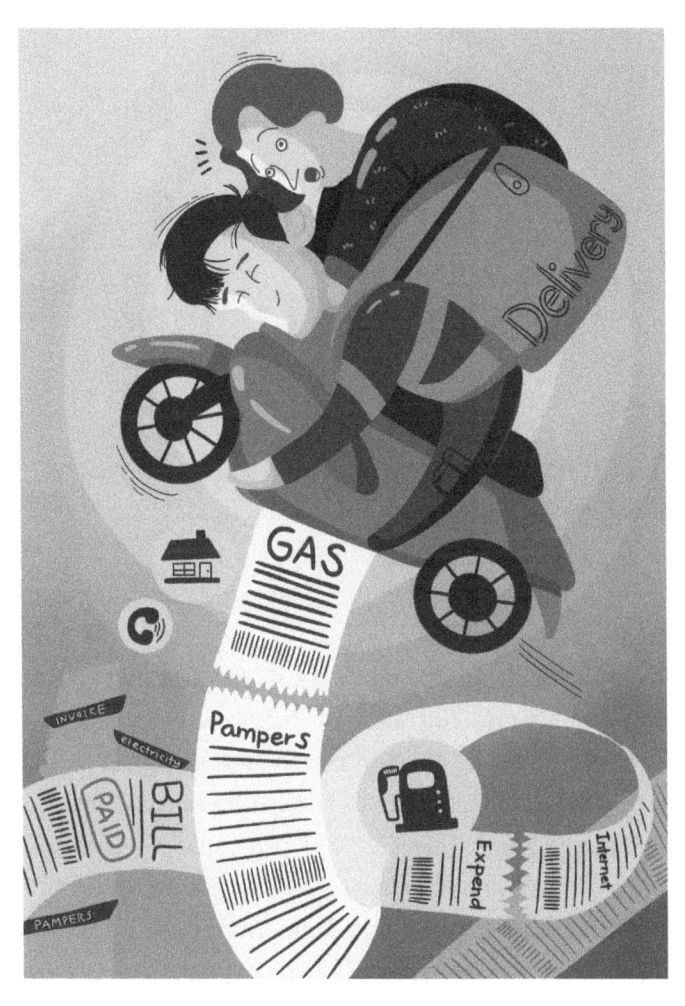

Illustrated by an artist who wishes to remain anonymous

STORY OF YAP

MENTAL WELLBEING

Sometime in 2021, my head started to feel tight as if it was being pulled from every direction. There was an ever-present high-pitched ringing in my ear. Unable to focus my thoughts or vision, I was in a persistent state of disorientation.

With each passing day, I felt more alone and unable to subdue a growing sense of inexplicable fear. I grew sensitive to noises coming from various corners of the flat. The bathroom was so frightfully noisy, I needed company to feel safe to use it. I also could not get close to the main door, which is a gateway to a cacophony of noises and other stimulants from unfamiliar sources.

Unable to leave the flat, I had to resign from my job as a specialist technician. I have worked at that shipyard for nearly thirty years, taking home a monthly salary of just over two thousand dollars. Looking back, there were some six years without a cent of a pay rise, and yet

I dutifully showed up for work each day. In recent years, there were only two of us from here and in our fifties, the rest of the workers are in their twenties and thirties and most of them come from India, Bangladesh, and Thailand. We pretty much kept to ourselves, plus there was no time to socialise at work.

My wife and sister kept asking me to seek medical help. It took some persuading but I finally agreed to see a doctor with my wife. That first visit led to repeated return visits as I was convinced that the medicines were exacerbating my anxieties. Each time, my wife has to apply for leave from her work as a cleaner to attend the appointments with me, and each time, the doctor would say the same thing: the medication can help but only if I took it as prescribed for some time.

It would remain a mystery as to what exactly triggered my anxiety attacks. All I knew was it felt like a weight had lifted off me when my stepson moved out. Everything about him had bothered me. Other than fiddling with his mobile phone, he did not do much else at home. He is overweight and often smelt bad as we did not have air-conditioning in our flat.

My wife and I met online. A widow with a teenage son, she was working in a factory in Ho Chi Minh City then. For the first two years of our long-distance relationship, I shuttled back and forth between Singapore and Vietnam. We decided to marry so she could move to Singapore and live with me. It took over a year after our marriage to complete the adoption papers and arrange for her son to move to Singapore. That was some four years ago, and he was 16 years old then. Those were happier times.

Now, I have a daily routine to tire myself out so that I could manage a few hours of sleep at night. In the morning, I will spend more than an hour on self-care: wiping my eyes and applying an ointment for dry eyes, and taking (too) many pills for high blood pressure and anxiety. After medication and breakfast, I will be adapting my technical skills to do minor repairs at home, from fixing the standing fan to patching up a punctured bicycle tyre. I like the sense of satisfaction and accomplishment I get from these activities. In the evening, if it does not rain, I will cycle to the Sembawang beach which is just some ten minutes away. The sea breeze does wonders for me. I relish the momentary sense of peace and clarity at the beach.

The next step for me is to muster up the motivation to find employment. I hope to first find part-time work that starts in the afternoon, so I can go to my regular medical appointments. I have some experience as a forklift driver, it is a simple job that I believe I can do.

Story by Lai-Yee

What happened in the Story of Yap?

Yap's story provides a personal account of his experience and struggle with anxiety, and the impact it had on his life. His physical and mental symptoms gradually impacted his daily routine, functioning and well-being, forced him to resign from his long-term job as a specialist technician, and eventually led him to seek medical help. Yap's wife had to accompany him to appointments, showcasing the importance of support systems when navigating mental health challenges.

Mental illness is often invisible and stigmatised in many parts of the world, and the stigma can create barriers to accessing care. Yap's initial reluctance to seek medical help is common among individuals struggling with mental health issues. Health and medical services for people living with mental illness can often also be underdeveloped, resulting in them being undiagnosed, underserved and untreated. If these people are left undiagnosed and untreated, mental health conditions can become chronic and debilitating, leading to functional decline and social isolation.

Yap's anxiety made it challenging for him to socialize or connect with his colleagues at work. The age gap between him and his younger colleagues, along with their different nationalities, may have contributed to it and led to a sense of isolation. Mental health issues can impact one's ability to form and maintain social connections, potentially exacerbating feelings of loneliness and disconnection.

After getting medical attention and treatment, Yap established a daily routine which includes self-care practices and coping strategies to manage his anxiety. The application of eye ointment, taking medication for high blood pressure and anxiety, and engaging in minor repairs at home provide him with a sense of satisfaction and accomplishment. These activities help Yap distract himself from anxious thoughts and find moments of peace and clarity.

Yap's story underscores the importance of recognizing and addressing mental health concerns early on, as untreated anxiety disorders can worsen over time. Fortunately, majority of mental health conditions are treatable, and there is a strong chance of making a full recovery. Now that he is better, Yap plans to find part-time employment to give himself flexibility to manage his medical needs and appointments. His desire to work and contribute to society is evident and admirable.

In many countries and cities, there is also increased recognition of the importance and rising incidence of mental health conditions, leading to more and sustained investments in the health and social care sector to develop mental health services and promote mental well-being. Yap's story also highlights the importance of flexible work arrangements and accommodations for individuals with mental health concerns.

Despite the challenges Yap faced, his story is also one of perseverance, resilience and hope. Many people living with mental health conditions have the potential for recovery with proper treatment and support.

Thinking about why people get sick

Yap's story highlights the intersection of mental health and employment. His struggle with anxiety ultimately led to his resignation from a long-term job, impacting his finances and sense of stability. Mental health issues can create barriers to employment, and the loss of income can further exacerbate stress and negatively affect overall health - this underscores the need for workplace mental health support. In your community, how does mental health issues intersect with employment opportunities?

Recognising that there is still significant lack of understanding and stigma surrounding people with mental health conditions, are we aware of certain vulnerable groups in our society who may be at risk of undetected and undiagnosed mental health conditions? What are the community and family members' perception of a person suffering from mental health conditions?

In many places, mental health services are underdeveloped. Are the mental health services in our community known and accessible to people living with or at risk of mental health conditions? Are these people able to access these services without fear of stigma, especially in small tightly knit communities?

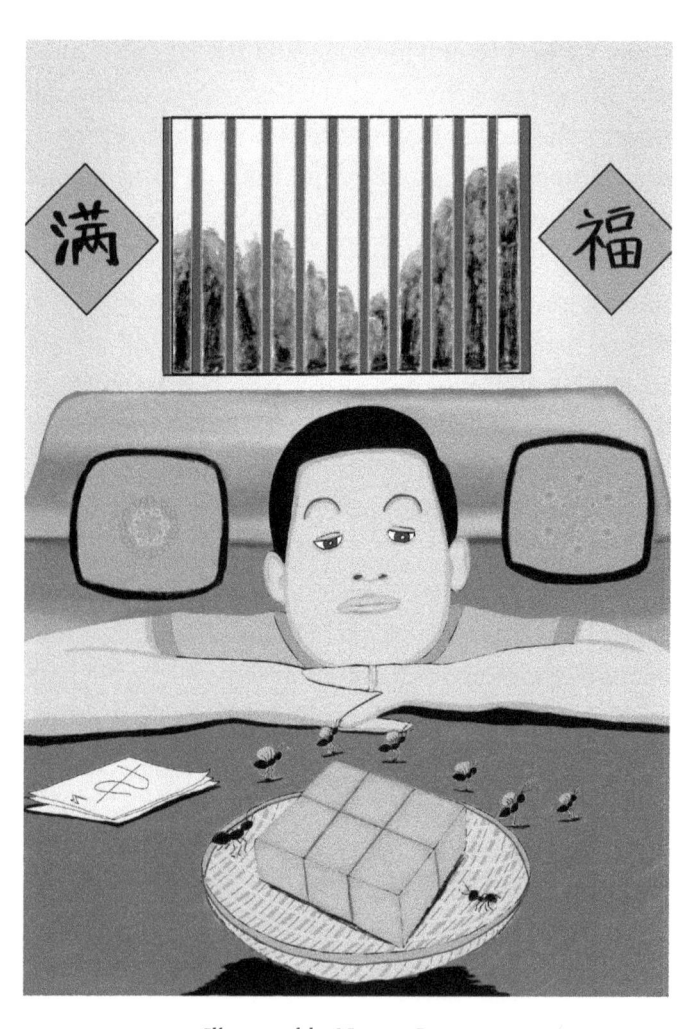

Illustrated by Norena Darsana
LinkedIn: linkedin.com/norena-darsana-885052164
Instagram: @northetutor

STORY OF JAMES

MAGNETIC

James always acted like a big bully at school. None of his classmates were safe from his tall shadow as he domineered his way through the hallways. No kid had the courage to stop James. Recently, he's been poking fun at Carlo, whom he called a sissy for carrying a pink bag at school.

One day, the class travelled to a nearby city for an art excursion. While viewing the exhibits, James saw what he thought was a very intriguing statue. It turns out that it wasn't a statue but a figure of a young man. James noticed this lad was glancing back at him, smiling. In response, James smirked and giggled, and couldn't resist whispering, "Ah, future husband of Carlo!" Then James ignored him and made his way through the museum.

Yet James was a bit intrigued. So he stayed in a corridor where he thought he might get another look at the guy. He took a deep breath and looked around.

Then, in the corridor, he saw the young man, a strong, fine figure, bearded, with toned arms. In his surprise, James rubbed his eyes to give him a second look. Seeing James, the man offered his hand for shake. James felt himself at a loss for words and melting to the charms of the young man – he's named Ian – and responded back with a fine grip of a handshake.

It turned out that Ian had spotted James when the group entered the museum, and started to approach and say "Hi..." when James had turned away. Their meeting in the museum turned into the beginning of a love story. While James acted like a bully, he was innocent about his sexuality. With Ian, James began trying to show his intimate feelings and exposing his vulnerabilities, as he learned what love was supposed to be.

Behind James' bullying attitude was a challenging childhood. He had been troubled by domestic abuse, and by sexual advances that he kept hidden behind his conscious memory. He had been in denial about his sexuality, and through his bullying he tried to make it clear to others that he was not attracted to boys. When he met Ian, James started to mellow, and he began sharing some of his hidden past with others.

However, as their relationship moved forward a few years, Ian began experiencing flashbacks and nightmares of his past, to the point that Ian took it as an opportunity to play around.

The adventures of Ian drastically affected James both mentally and physically. He was caught unaware when he learned that he had been infected, and was living with asymptomatic infections brought by multiple partners of Ian. James spent his years in paranoia, never trying to make friends with other men for the fear of liking them. In the past, he had used his bullying to hide his sexuality. Now he started dating women, and bragging about his dating escapades.

One day, he found himself alone in his apartment, drugged and lying naked on the floor. He was in an extreme state of depression. Struggling for his sanity and life, he grabbed the sink, pulled himself up, and faced the cracked mirror before him. Gazing into the mirror, he saw the familiar face of a man staring back at him, and he said, "Yes, it is I. At last, we meet."

Story by Jose Augustus VILLANO

What happened in the Story of James?

James' story is a complex narrative that explores themes of bullying, self-discovery, and the impact of past trauma on mental health.

James' bullying behaviour is revealed to be a coping mechanism for his own internal struggles and trauma. The intersection of bullying and mental health highlights how individuals may act out as a way to cope with pain, confusion, or denial about their true self. James' denial about his sexuality and internalized homophobia contribute to his aggressive behavior as a means of projecting an image of heterosexual masculinity.

James' self-discovery journey intersects with his mental health and well-being. The process of accepting his true sexuality involves confronting internalized stigma and societal expectations. The fear of rejection and discrimination can lead to self-concealment, isolation, and mental health struggles.

James' challenging childhood, marked by domestic abuse and sexual advances, has left deep scars. Past trauma can increase the risk of mental health issues, including depression, anxiety, and post-traumatic stress disorder (PTSD). The intersection of trauma and mental health highlights how adverse experiences can shape an individual's behavior, relationships, and overall well-being.

The dynamic between James and Ian underscores the impact of romantic relationships on mental health. Unhealthy relationship dynamics, such as infidelity and emotional manipulation, can exacerbate mental health struggles. Ian's behavior triggers flashbacks and nightmares for James, affecting him mentally and physically. This aspect of the story emphasizes the importance of mutual support, trust, and healthy relationship dynamics for positive mental health outcomes.

The discovery of James' sexually transmitted infection (STI) highlights the intersection of sexual health and mental health. The stigma associated with and lack of understanding of sexually transmitted infections can lead to self-blame, isolation, and paranoia, delayed treatment, increased risk behaviours, and poorer mental health outcomes. James' response to his STI diagnosis is to isolate himself and engage in risky behaviours. Isolation and self-blame are common responses to a newly discovered STI diagnosis due to internalized shame and fear of rejection.

The conclusion of the story, with James facing depression and suicidal ideation, underscores the seriousness of mental health issues and the need for early recognition and timely intervention to prevent tragic outcomes. But the image of James confronting his reflection in the mirror could also symbolize self-reflection and the potential for positive change. We hope that James is able face his past trauma, accept his sexuality, and acknowledge his true self. Self-acceptance and self-compassion are vital steps toward the promise of healing, rebuilding self-worth and one's resilience.

Thinking about why people get sick

James' story provides insight into the complex interplay and dynamics between bullying, self-discovery, internal struggles, past trauma, mental health, and sexual health. His story also illuminates health inequities influenced by social determinants. The lack of supportive environments for self-exploration and the impact of past trauma contribute to poorer mental health outcomes. Additionally, the stigma associated with STIs and the lack of sexual health education in marginalised and vulnerable communities can result in delayed treatment and increased mental health burdens.

Reflecting on James' bullying behaviour and the possible underlying causes and environmental factors, how does our community perceive bullying behaviours of adolescents and youths? Do people understand the potential impact of bullying on the mental health and wellbeing of both the bully and the bullied?

While it is not easy to unpack why people bully others, we can see that for James it could have resulted from his challenging childhood. Do people in our community understand the potential long-term effects of childhood trauma on mental health outcomes and recognise the need for early intervention?

For James, his unhealthy relationship dynamics with Ian, which includes infidelity and emotional manipulation, can exacerbate James' mental health struggles. In our communities, do people understand that unhealthy relationship dynamics can negatively impact mental well-being? How does the community show empathy and support these persons?

The mental health implications and the associated stigma of a new STI diagnosis can be difficult to manage, especially in tight-knit communities where news travel fast. An environment where diagnosis is hidden and not communicated, can lead to delayed treatment and poor health outcomes. In our community, are people similarly afraid to come forward to share their diagnosis and seek treatment?

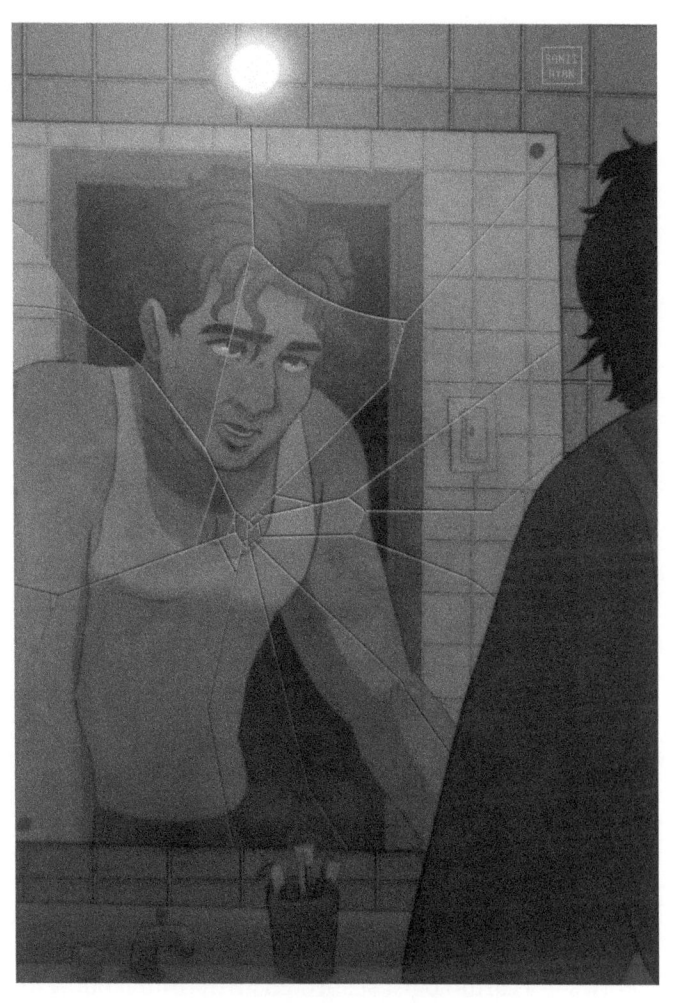

Illustrated by SK Kapangyarihan
X and Instagram: @samiihyan

STORY OF AFINA

EPILEPSY

At eight years old, I confided in my mother about my headaches, but she dismissed them as my imagination, claiming a child couldn't have one-sided headaches. "You're just imitating those painkiller ads!" she said, shutting down my pain. From then on, I endured sleep difficulties, becoming a light sleeper easily awakened by the slightest noise.

Later, when I was in high school, I would frequently drift into a dreamlike state before succumbing to sudden unconsciousness. Fainting episodes plagued my days, disrupting my education and incurring complaints from teachers and peers. Countless doctors offered divergent theories—a cardiologist suspected arrhythmia, but tests proved inconclusive. A neurologist finally unveiled a specific diagnosis: atonic epilepsy.

The diagnosis validated my complaints, but it also opened a Pandora's box. My mother, told the neurologist: "Someone from her paternal family had Stevens-Johnson syndrome." Stevens-Johnson syndrome is a severe form of hypersensitivity reaction, and while considered a rare health condition, it is prevalent among East and Southeast Asians. I was still in shock, digesting the diagnosis. I did understand, though, that the neurologist was concerned about giving me the standard epilepsy medications. Instead, he prescribed the minimum treatment dose of another drug he judged less dangerous to my body, considering my risk for the syndrome.

Unfortunately, I experienced strange side effects from the drug. My muscles were naturally weak due to epilepsy, so I could easily fall or faint. The drug made my muscles stiffen and, on several occasions, even moved my joints — my arms could suddenly shake and move on their own. It was terrifying. I was forced to stop the drug after only a short period.

Without medication, I focused on trigger management for my epilepsy, avoiding hot weather, sun, fatigue, stress, and certain foods. Processed foods became a thing of the past as my body craved low-carb, low-sugar options. Seeking alternatives, my parents took me to a renowned healer who provided herbal medicine from noni fruit extract and honey. After a year of this regimen, my condition improved, and I no longer experienced fainting episodes.

Yet the weight of secrecy and the complexity of treatment persisted. No one, not even my sibling or boyfriend, was entrusted with this secret. I felt ashamed and believed that epilepsy was something to be hidden, allowing others to perceive me simply as naturally weak. A haunting memory from my childhood reinforced these fears. I had witnessed a man collapsing on the road, his body convulsing, frothy drool escaping his mouth. Surrounding onlookers did nothing, warning against contact with his saliva and suggesting futile remedies. Having witnessed that scene, I felt that it made sense when my parents urged me to keep my epilepsy a secret.

Epilepsy leaves me vulnerable, and a traumatic event I experienced more than 10 years ago made my vulnerability very clear. While in the sweltering heat of Yogyakarta, I succumbed to disorientation and unease. I experienced sexual assault at that time, when I was unconscious. The memory of that attack still lingers, shaping my cautious steps through the streets, wary of whom I trust and where I find myself. The fear of manipulation looms, a reminder that those with hidden intentions can shatter trust. Remaining single became a choice born out of a lack of trust, as society deems women like me unworthy of unconditional love. Witnessing husbands abandon their sick wives in my community also reinforced this belief.

Over the years, I have explored many treatments to try to stabilize my condition. I have followed a strict diet, I have tried herbal remedies, and I have found solace in online epilepsy support groups. I have tried combinations of medication, but have experienced side effects, and one drug triggered Stevens-Johnson syndrome. Half a year ago, I decided to leave my job in Jakarta for a more peaceful environment in Yogyakarta. I have found some relief in this world away from Jakarta, and in detaching myself from what is "modern," but it comes at a cost.

I do understand that epilepsy cannot be cured. But I want to manage it to have better quality of life even though I live with epilepsy. My health journey is complex, intertwining physical, emotional, and societal dimensions. Yet I refuse to let other people's perceptions define me, understanding that centuries of stigma cannot dictate my worth.

For people like me, the reality of being chronically ill shapes our lives and experiences. Sadly, our rhythm often clashes with a world that fails to understand. I don't have all the answers, but I know we deserve better than being treated as second-class with limited choices. By sharing our stories, we can challenge long-standing stigmas surrounding chronic illnesses. We can create an environment where stereotypes crumble and collective healing becomes a reality – a vision free from the unwarranted shame we never deserve to bear.

Story by Afina

What happened in the Story of Afina?

Afina's story offers a personal account of living with epilepsy, navigating treatment options, and the impact of stigma on the individual's experiences. Afina's early experiences of headaches and sleep difficulties were dismissed by her mother as imaginary and may reflect a lack of understanding. These responses may contribute to Afina's feelings of isolation and even shame, as she tries to navigate fainting episodes during her school years, which disrupted her education and led to feedback from her teachers.

It was hard for Afina to get her condition correctly diagnosed, she had to consult with multiple doctors and specialists. Even when Afina was diagnosed with epilepsy, her diagnosis is kept secret, even from siblings and boyfriend. This secrecy is influenced by the stigma associated with epilepsy in her socio-cultural context, and the fear of being perceived as weak or abnormal. Afina's recollection of a memory of a man experiencing a seizure on the road and the lack of assistance from surrounding onlookers reinforces her fear. The internalized shame and fear of rejection that leads to Afina concealing her condition can negatively impacting her social interactions and relationships.

Afina's treatment journey involves a complex interplay of western medications, alternative treatments, and lifestyle changes. The decision to leave her job in Jakarta for a more peaceful environment reflects Afina's maturity and recognition that epilepsy is a life-long condition. Her move to Yogyakarta reflects her desire for a more peaceful environment that supports her health needs and journey to recovery.

Afina's experiences highlight the need for awareness and understanding to create supportive environments for individuals with epilepsy.

Thinking about why people get sick

Epilepsy can significantly impact a person's ability to attend school or work regularly, participate in social activities, and maintain relationships. In your community, how does stigma associated with epilepsy impact individuals and their experiences in the community?

From Afina's story we can experience the emotional and social dimensions of a person living with epilepsy, and highlights the intersection of epilepsy and stigma. We can see how societal misconceptions and misunderstandings can impact an individual's experiences with epilepsy, a life-long and chronic illness. Her experiences of secrecy, stigma, and the traumatic event of sexual assault affect her worldview, sense of self-worth and outlook on life, and can lead to poorer health outcomes. Do you know of people living with epilepsy in your community, and in what ways can stigma lead to social isolation and poorer health outcomes in the long-term?

In certain situations where epilepsy can negatively affect an individual's ability to attend school or work regularly – could that lead to other medical conditions like depression or unhealthy habits like smoking or alcohol? For people living with epilepsy and are on medications, how do you think the side effects of the medication can influence their quality of life?

In the management and treatment of a person's epilepsy, the lack of a strong supportive environment and timely access to health services can lead to non-compliance, a sense of fatalism and loss of hope, and even substance abuse – leading to a downward spiral of poor health outcomes.

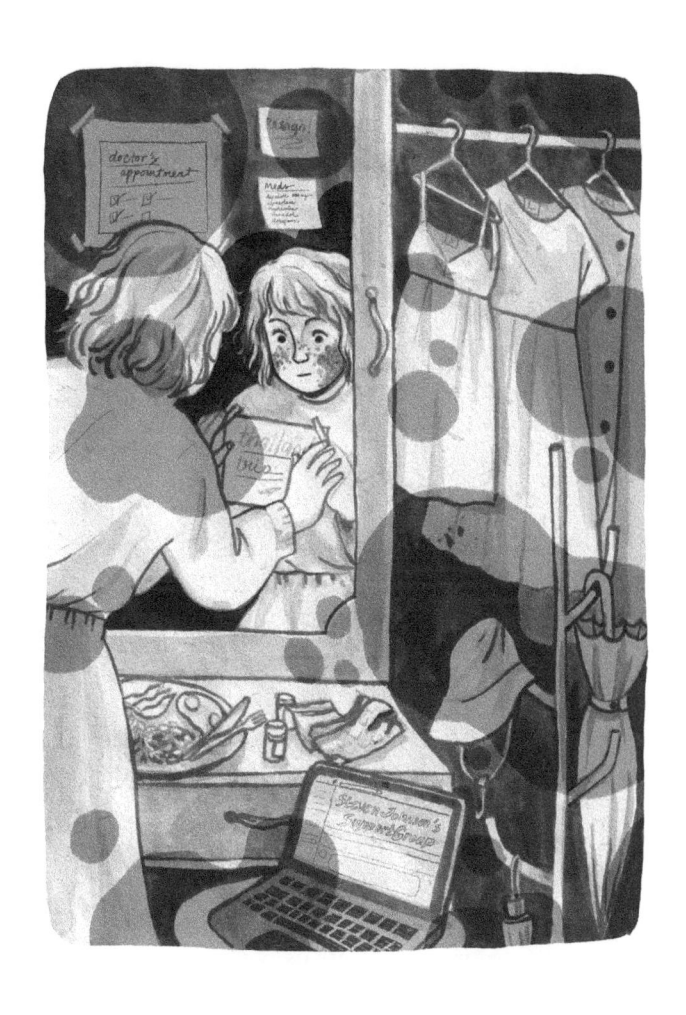

Illustrated by Nadiyah Suyatna
nadiyahsuyatna.com

STORY OF SUPAP

POLLUTION

I recall the days when Wisan and I toiled under the hot sun in the fields of Huai Lek ravine. Those fields weren't always filled with what we see now - rambutans and lychees. They were once lush rice paddies, tended to by my forefathers before us. But life has a way of changing, and so did our fields.

Our journey back to the countryside from bustling Bangkok was born out of need and a sense of responsibility. In 2003, we received the news that my parents had passed away. It was then that we knew we had to return, to tend to the land they cherished, the legacy and memories they left us with.

My mother, before she passed away, fought valiantly against the environmental destruction caused by mining activities. She wrote letters and travelled by public bus to submit those letters to the government officials, to tell them about the damaged fields resulting from the mineral exploitation. Although a government agency intervened by excavating the topsoil and filling the affected land, the rice plants remained damaged, and their growth affected - the damage to our rice fields was irreparable.

The effects of the mining operations extended beyond the fields and into our home. We witnessed the inexplicable loss of loved ones, one after another, to mysterious illnesses. My father, once strong and resilient, succumbed to a sudden fever accompanied by blackening and stiffening of the skin. He died in 2003 at the young age of 56. The doctors labelled it a heart attack, but it felt like so much more. Then, just months later in the same year, my mother also died suddenly, with similar signs and symptoms. They said it was liver cancer, but I couldn't shake the feeling that it was something connected to the environmental damage of the land.

Even my dear grandfather, a pillar of strength in our family, died at the age of 77 – suffering from the same signs and symptoms as my father and mother. In his death certificate – the cause of death was written as cancer.

The land, once rich with life, became a wasteland. My family had relied upon rice cultivation in the Huay Lek Creek for our livelihood, gathering vegetables, and using the shallow wells in the fields for food, drinking water, and irrigation. I clearly remember the day when the provincial public health department issued a warning regarding the consumption of water, aquatic animals, and vegetables from Huay Lek Creek. They said there was unsafe levels of heavy metal substances, specifically arsenic contamination, in the water. We could no longer use water from the creek and cultivate rice, and could not use the land for over a decade.

Our family had to suffer the harmful consequences and legacy of this gold mining site in Khao Luang sub-district, Wang Saphung District, Loei Province, located in the northeast of Thailand. Our communities living in the areas surrounding the mine have been engaged in an intense struggle for environmental justice for many years. We had successfully campaigned for the permanent closure of the gold mine and demanded action from both the company and the Thai government to address social, ecological, and health restoration. A court judgment found that gold mining operations resulted in contamination to surrounding regions, with the spread of heavy metals such as arsenic, manganese, iron, lead, mercury, and other toxins. The contamination significantly our villagers' livelihoods, causing harm to people's lives, bodies, health, and mental well-being. The closure of the gold mine brought little solace to our grieving community. The scars it left behind were deep and lasting, a constant reminder of the environmental devastation and its impact on the communities in the area.

While the mine has been closed since 2013, our struggle for environmental justice is not over. A court ruled that the mining company had a duty to restore the environment, but the company has since gone bankrupt.

Our community members want to be involved in restoration planning and rehabilitation operations, but negotiations with government agencies to accept community participation are taking a long time.

Nevertheless, our community remains determined and united to continue the social, ecological and health restoration efforts of the area, to restore the environment, one step at a time.

Story by Bampen Chaiyarak

What happened in the Story of Supap?

Supap's story sheds light on the devastating impact of environmental injustice and the resilience of communities fighting for environmental and health restoration.

Supap's community has suffered the consequences of gold mining activities in their region, specifically the contamination of heavy metals like arsenic, manganese, iron, lead, and mercury. The narrative highlights how environmental injustice, particularly the contamination of water and soil, can have direct health impacts on communities. Supap's family experienced sudden deaths and illnesses, with symptoms like high fever, skin discoloration, and organ failure, ultimately leading to cancer and heart attacks.

The contamination of the rice fields and water sources resulted in the loss of Supap's family livelihood and food security. Their reliance on rice cultivation and the use of water from the creek for food and irrigation were abruptly disrupted. The warning from the public health department about unsafe levels of heavy metal substances forced them to cease their agricultural activities, creating economic hardship and uncertainty.

The health impacts of environmental injustice are felt across generations. Supap's parents, grandparents, and several family members experienced illnesses and deaths due to the contamination. From Supap's story we can see how environmental injustices can have long-lasting consequences, affecting not only the immediate community but also future generations.

Supap's community has displayed remarkable resilience and advocacy in their fight for environmental and health restoration. They successfully campaigned for the permanent closure of the gold mine and they shared a strong determination to address the social, ecological, and health impacts of environmental injustice. We see the power of community advocacy in demanding accountability, seeking justice, and influencing policy changes to prevent future environmental harms.

Thinking about why people get sick

The health impacts of environmental injustice can have long-term effects, requiring ongoing health monitoring. Communities living in polluted areas may face increased risks of cancer, cardiovascular diseases, respiratory issues, and other health concerns due to their exposure to toxins. This highlights the importance of social determinants of health – conditions in which people are born, grow, live, work, and age – in influencing and impact health outcomes. Through Supap's story, we can see the direct connection between environmental injustice, loss of livelihoods and health inequities – and the intersection between environmental injustice, health impacts, community resilience, and the ongoing struggle for justice and restoration.

In our community, how do environmental pollution and injustice contribute to health inequities? Do we see situations where environmental pollution and injustices disrupt people's livelihoods and affect their health status?

Are our communities concerned about the potential health risks faced by future generations due environmental pollution leading to early life exposures to toxins and heavy metals?

How can communities come together and organise themselves to be heard and to advocate for their right to a healthy living environment?

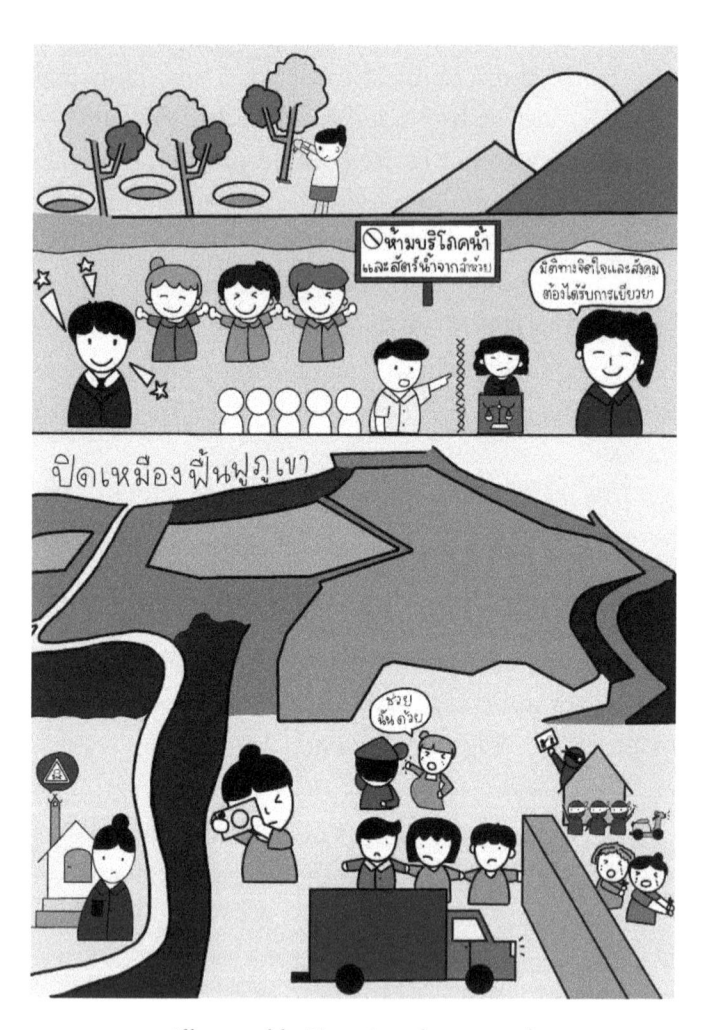

Illustrated by Tana Aeambumrungsub
Instagram: @tanaceleb

STORY OF ROSA

GEOGRAPHY

In 2019, someone I know very well started having a mental health problem. At that time, we did not realize what that actually was. He would be talking like a drunk for a couple of days straight, not sleeping. It was more than a little chaos. He is a leader, someone who always has my back and is smart. I was sad and shocked but at the same time forced myself to appear emotionless because who then will be in charge? Family asked for advice from people, going from one place to another looking for traditional healers – four in total, from west to east of our regency. Nothing changed. Making them bring him to the hospital was a struggle. They still tended to go to traditional healers or religious leaders.

In my community, some people prefer home treatment to getting a doctor's prescription. Going to a medical provider is often seen as only for very bad or chronic diseases. Even though people have access to education and are supposedly aware of the benefits of modern medicine, they still strongly adhere to traditional beliefs. For example, among the local tribes and community, there is a general belief that people become sick because of other people's evildoing or an evil spirit. One way to heal the ailments caused by those things, according to the belief, is by consulting a traditional healer and practicing certain ceremonies, or by consulting certain people who are deemed as more spiritual, asking for their prayers and healing potions. This still happens. For every five sick people I know, three would go for traditional medicine. Sometimes it is an individual's decision. At other times, it is the family's or the community's.

However, I kept pushing for the person I know to see a doctor. I felt like I was the only one who was aware of what could go wrong. Looking back, I honestly cannot imagine what would happen if we only did things the traditional way. But the path to treatment was not easy. There were no mental health services at the hospital on our island in 2021 and it is not even common yet. We had to go to another regency for diagnosis and treatment. We had to wait a long time when we arrived, as the staff who usually helped the doctor was not there. Then, we were given antipsychotic medications without proper understanding about them. Still, the treatment helped. He got better and we thought that was the happy ending. We let him be, not bringing him for further consultation, because he actually seemed better. Besides, the psychiatrist's place was too far. We did not discuss the condition further or look for more information.

I did not know about the possibility of relapse so I thought that our nightmare was over. But in 2023, he had another psychotic episode. Fortunately, this time we could access the medications at the nearby *Puskesmas* (a community health centre) and then got referred for therapy at a clinic nearby. We were finally able to create a very supportive environment for him, including making sure he gets and takes his medications. I do wish that our experience with the previous doctor's communication had been better. There was not enough explanation about what was happening, and we were not aware that if we stop the medications, there will be a possibility of relapse.

I have kept looking to have the best service at the best price that seems fair for everyone including patients and psychiatric. I am still angry about the price, and I still demand cheaper treatment and comparable services in our areas compared to nearby regency. It seems due to the distance and distribution as well as the minimum number of services. I know that there are other neighbours who are not able to pay or to access information.

My experience is not unique. In fact, similar problems happen quite frequently, either because of late treatment or poor awareness of the early symptoms. There are so many reasons for this: cultural barriers, socio-economic status, lifestyle, and others. I somehow have mixed feelings, sad, worried, relieved but angry for unfairness to access. Reflecting on those days, I was able to carry on thanks to my colleagues who have given continuous support in time and mental health information. It was difficult to open up but things were getting clear and I gained more strength.

It was frustrating as well because at some point it seemed like they found it easier to blame other people for bad things happening in the family rather than acknowledge that their loved one was actually sick. I kept pushing. Then we finally reached an agreement to do both approaches, medical and traditional. Looking back, I honestly cannot imagine what would happen if we only did things the traditional way.

Access to healthcare can have a different meaning in rural areas than in urban areas. It's a life journey in advocating fairness in both areas, adapting to each of the characteristics. The sadness and anger I had gave me a voice to say that other family should face the same situation, because it's a painful journey to compare what access you could not get just because you stay in a rural area.

Story by Rosadalima Dee PANDA

What happened in the Story of Rosa?

The Indonesian government provides free healthcare for communities through the "Indonesian Health Card", introduced in 2014. This programme helps the vulnerable community and individuals access care regardless of their background and ability to pay. However in rural communities, like the one in the story, people often face challenges such as limited mental health services, limited access to psychotropic medications, longer travel distances to access care, fewer specialized care providers, and reduced availability of crisis intervention services. These disparities contribute to treatment delays and potentially poorer health outcomes. These health services disparities have the potential to reinforce social and economic inequalities, impacting vulnerable communities disproportionately.

The difficulty in accessing these mental healthcare services may lead to the rural communities turning to traditional healing methods, which is also deeply rooted in cultural beliefs and practices. While traditional practices can provide comfort and cultural meaning, relying solely on them for severe mental health issues may potentially lead to inadequate treatment. As a result, rural community may tend to view mental health issues as something to be addressed only when they become severe. This delay in seeking professional help can result in a more complex treatment journey and potentially poorer health outcomes. The intersection of cultural beliefs and healthcare access highlights the need for culturally sensitive and responsive mental healthcare services.

The story above also highlights that the narrator, as a caregiver, can also experience a range of emotions and struggle with their own mental well-being. Caregivers of individuals with mental illness often face caregiver burden and secondary traumatization. The lack of support systems and mental health literacy in rural areas can isolate caregivers, impacting their ability to provide effective care and support.

Thinking about why people get sick

Rosa's story provide a glimpse into how rural communities may have difficulties in accessing specialized medical services. Think about a rural community or a person living in a difficult to access area, how do healthcare disparities manifest because of these access challenges? Do you think there are significant differences when it comes to treatment pathways between rural and urban communities? What are some of the potential financial challenges faced by individuals in rural areas when seeking specialised mental healthcare services?

In Rosa's story, we are shown the difficulties encountered when navigating mental healthcare access for their loved one. What are the additional burdens and difficulties for caregivers living in rural areas? What unique challenges do caregivers in rural areas face? How does isolation based on geography impact caregivers and their ability to care for their loved ones and themselves? How can communities support and advocate for rural caregivers?

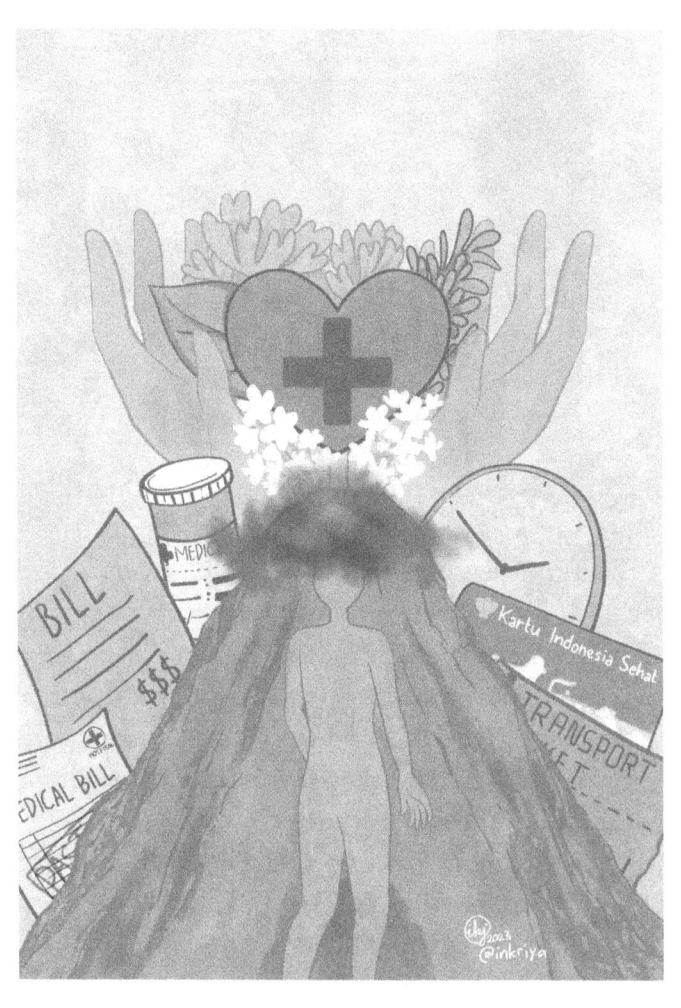

Illustrated by Inez Kriya
X: @by_inkriya | Instagram: @inkriya

STORY OF THERESA

CONFLICT

My name is Naw Teresa. I am 25 years old and from Myanmar. I have four sisters and five brothers. To support us when we were children, my parents had to pick dog fruit, a fruit that villagers normally eat with rice. To cover the annual school fees for one child, it took them two days to pick two full packs of dog fruit in the jungle. Then they had to walk for a whole day to arrive at the river and then ride a boat for two hours to sell the fruit in town.

That meant my parents could not afford to pay for all of us to go to school. They could only send three daughters to the only primary school in my village. Meanwhile, my eldest brother had to babysit my younger siblings.

Due to my parents' selfless sacrifice, I was able to go to school until second grade. After second grade, I had to go to another village and stay with my aunt to continue with third grade, as my parents could not support me anymore. Becoming a teacher was my dream, and I hoped that someday I could provide free education to children who could not afford the school fee.

I was fortunate to continue my studying from grades four to ten, and then I joined the Leadership and Management Training College. After finishing, I contributed my knowledge as a high school teacher for two years. Then, since I am passionate about promoting local income generation, I applied for a scholarship and got the chance to study social business and organizational development.

After I finished my academic program in early 2021, I went back to my village. Soon after, my family faced a horrible thing. My elder brother, who was the breadwinner of our family, was killed by the military in March, one month after the military coup. Consequently, both of my parents' mental health deteriorated, so I decided to stay with them.

However, my father encouraged me to look beyond current obstacles and contribute to the community. Many people were suffering and having a hard time, and children were not able to access education due to prolonged conflicts. I was approached by the local education committee to teach at the middle school, and I pushed myself to overcome my fear and start working as a schoolteacher. It was the only middle school for seven villages, and there were a total of 115 students from kindergarten to grade nine. There are 12 teachers that work closely with the school committee to make sure that school is functioning and students are progressing during this very challenging time.

Our school was not safe from conflict. The school, clinics, churches, houses, and other buildings were bombed by the military junta's airstrikes. Two members of the school committee were killed by shelling, and more children became orphans. All the women, children, and elderly hide in the jungle with limited rations and nutritional support. Access to basic health care needs is a real challenge. Children's mental health is in critical need of healing. Teachers and school committees are overburdened with emergency response, school property maintenance, and children's safety in low-resource situations. Nutritional assistance, clean water, and mobile sanitary toilets are critical needs in the current situation.

Due to this crisis situation, several non-local teachers have terminated their volunteering at our school. That means there are only six local teachers left to run the school next year. As our Plan B, we will prepare temporary learning shelters in the jungle, where we will teach the students until the situation gets a bit stable. As these villages are not close to each other or to our current temporary shelter, every year we prepare a dormitory shelter for the students. This year we might face more challenges since our existing resources are very limited and there will not be much support available from the central Karen Education and Culture Department since many schools are in need of essential support.

However, I do not give up. I try to read whenever I get a chance, so that I can continue to contribute to the promotion of education and resilience in the jungle.

Story by Naw Pue Pue Mhote

What happened in the Story of Theresa?

Naw Teresa's story provides a powerful account of resilience, dedication to education, and the impact of conflict on access to education and healthcare for people living in conflict zones.

The conflict has disrupted access to basic needs such as nutrition, clean water, and sanitation. Nutritional assistance, mobile sanitary toilets, and access to healthcare are critical needs in the current situation. Conflict and violence often result in the destruction of infrastructure and essential services, impacting the overall health and well-being of the community.

The school and surrounding areas are not immune to the conflict. Airstrikes, shelling, and violence affect the school, clinics, places of worship, and residential areas. The loss of lives, including members of the school committee, and the displacement of families puts a spotlight on the direct impact of conflict on access to education and healthcare. In these conflict zones, there are concerns about the children's mental health and overall well-being, and also how teachers and school committees are overburdened, both mentally and physically, with teaching duties, emergency response and ensuring students' safety.

In conflict zones, the long-term impact on children's mental health may not be highlighted. But we know that conflict, violence, displacement, and the loss of loved ones take a significant toll on the mental health and emotional well-being of children. We also recognise the bravery and dedication of community members like Naw Teresa, who have dedicated their time and life to teaching and supporting children's education and mental health in the midst of conflict, even if it means putting themselves in danger.

Naw Teresa's story takes a tragic turn with the death of her elder brother due to the military coup. This loss not only affects the family financially but also takes an emotional toll, particularly on her parents, whose mental health deteriorates. Conflict and violence have direct and indirect impacts on the well-being of individuals and communities, often disrupting access to education and essential services.

Despite the immense challenges, Naw Teresa remains hopeful and dedicated to her mission. She continues to pursue her passion for promoting education and resilience, even in the face of adversity. Her commitment to reading and self-improvement perhaps highlights her belief in the transformative power of education and self-improvement. Her resilience and determination to overcome obstacles are inspiring and reflect her unwavering commitment to her community and the strength of the human spirit.

Thinking about why people get sick

Despite her own challenges, Naw Teresa decides to stay and contribute to her community. She answers the call to teach at the local middle school, which serves seven villages. Her dedication to education and the well-being of children in the midst of conflict is admirable. Naw Teresa's resilience and commitment to promoting education in challenging circumstances are testament to her character and sense of duty.

Looking at this story from an intersectional lens, we can gain a deeper understanding of the complex dynamics between poverty, conflict, community resilience, and the fundamental right to education and healthcare.

From Naw Teresa's story, we can reflect on what the circumstances and living conditions of people living in conflict zones and how they have limited access to healthcare and education. What are the other basic infrastructure and essential services that can be disrupted that will cause these people living in conflict zones to have poorer health outcomes?

Considering the children highlighted in Naw Teresa's story, what are the specific mental health needs of children that may be areas of concern in the near term? What are some of the potential long-term effects of conflict, violence, and displacement on children's emotional well-being and their ability to cope with future challenges?

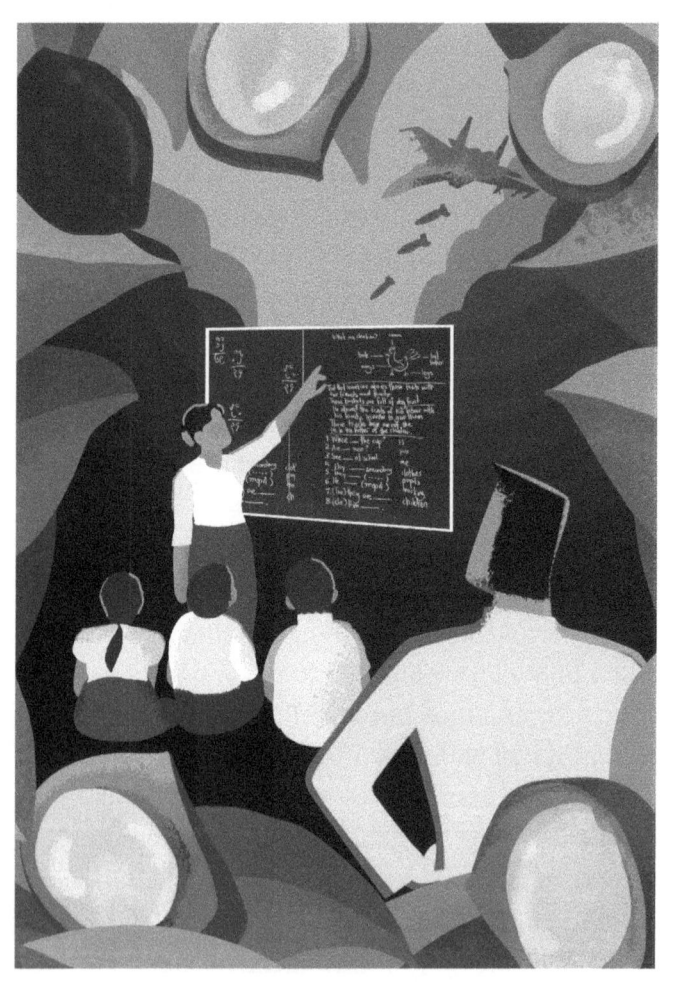

Illustrated by Khin Thawdar Khine
kaisauce.myportfolio.com

ABOUT THE EDITORS

Clive TAN is a medical doctor and a public health specialist. He's also an explorer, a teacher, a researcher, a daydreamer, a doer, a writer, a poet, a husband, and a father to three – Alexis, Matthias, and Avery. He's a left brainer who's discovering his right brain, and is fascinated by architecture's duality, and wishes to learn more about how architecture can be applied to imagine and build better health systems of the future.

Putri Widi SARASWATI (they/she) is an Indonesian intersectional feminist, a global public health specialist, and a medical doctor. One of their biggest dreams is to contribute to the integration of intersectional feminist perspective into shaping health – including the recognition of power dynamics that can determine one's health status and access to care, and by actively tackling inequity created by imbalance of power relations in the health sector. They are also a convener and collaborator for matters related to social justice and global health equity, celebrating equitable collaboration more than competition.

Eaint Thiri THU is a researcher, fixer and documentary producer specialized in conflicts and human rights in Myanmar. She is also a storyteller, dancer, calligrapher and restaurant owner. Growing up in the conflict society and under military dictatorship, she believes that hope, imagination and dedication are pivots to create a better system in the future.

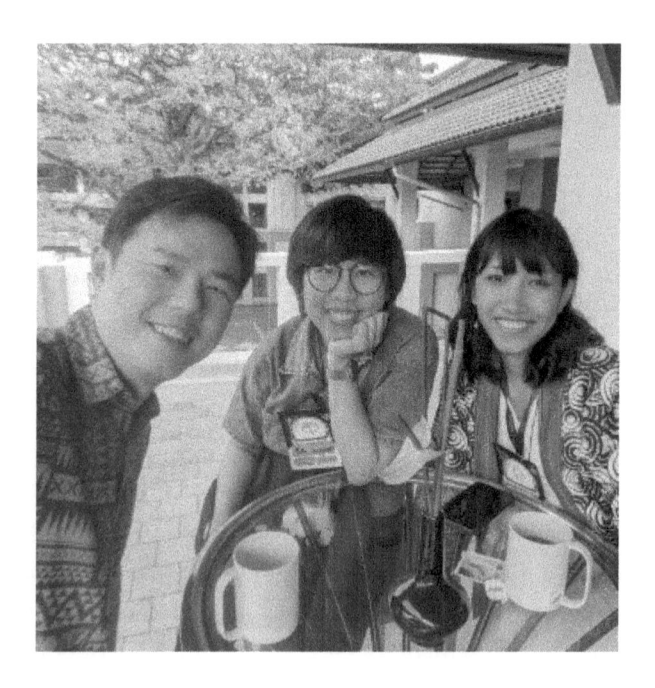

ABOUT THE WRITERS

Lena is a wife and a dog mom to 2 skittish mongrels and a stubborn dachshund. She is also a community health social worker who believes in Mother Teresa's quote: "Not all of us can do great things, but we can do small things with great love". Therefore, she is dedicated in using her limited capabilities to help people get through difficult situations, integrate them into their communities, and empower their way to physical, mental, and emotional recovery.

Lai-Yee has held roles in intergovernmental, non-profit, and charitable organisations, as well as the corporate sector. She champions inclusion, access, and sustainable empowerment for communities placed at-risk or disadvantaged in her professional and volunteering efforts. From healthcare to education, social entrepreneurship to culture, she is building multisectoral partnerships, impactful programmes and philanthropy, international networks, and effective teams.

Katie Kanyarat FERGUSON shared this about herself: "I am dedicated to producing valuable content alongside my team in order to contribute to society by enhancing individuals' physical and mental well-being, ultimately improving their quality of life. I find great satisfaction in collaborating with healthcare professionals and providing education and assistance to individuals, enabling them to take proactive measures in self-care and minimize their reliance on doctors and hospitals whenever possible."

Jun LAU is an avid learner and believes that good design can impact communities for good. Her practice in Organisation Development and Design Research has helped her to harness the power of observation and co-create solutions, with a diverse group of people, to address social issues. Apart from work, Jun enjoys walking barefoot in the park on a sunny day and making sourdough bread for her family and friends.

"Agah" Jose Augustus VILLANO is an experienced public servant in the Philippines with over a decade of experience across public and private sectors. He enjoys writing short notes and scribbles as a hobby. Professionally, he crafts policy recommendations and spearheads projects to meet his constituents' needs. With expertise in community medicine, economics, and law, he identifies vulnerable populations and advises on regional policy and resource allocation. Proudly, he's also a fur dad to eight delightful felines.

Collins SANTHANASAMY is a medical doctor from Malaysia with over a decade of field experience in South and Southeast Asia. His work with urban poor, refugee and rural communities focuses on the development of innovative and sustainable solutions that address the challenges of health, education and economic empowerment. He is passionate about Disaster Risk Reduction (DRR) and building community resilience.

ZHOU Haibin is a social entrepreneur and standards-based business and human rights, diversity and equality professional, with extensive experiences of working in China. He has extensive experiences at design, management, implementation, monitoring, and evaluation of multiple partners programs. Haibin is skilled at social development, sustainability, legal, human rights and policy advocacy, especially strong in Cooperate Social Responsibility, supply chains, labor law and equality issues.

Afina Nurul Faizah is a dedicated Reproductive Justice Advocate with extensive experience in social safeguards, gender mainstreaming, and policy development. She has worked on various projects related to human rights and minority issues, with a particular focus on advocating for the rights and well-being of women and marginalized communities in Southeast Asia.

Bampen CHAIYARAK is a writer focusing on cultures, nature, and human interactions. Her work emphasises social-ecological systems and health equity, drawing from her extensive fieldwork to author many non-fiction documentary books and in-depth reports. She's also the Co-founder and Coordinator for the project for Building Restorative Culture Coalition Thailand (RCCT).

Rosadalima Dee PANDA is born and raised in Flores East Nusa Tenggara Timur, Indonesia. She has working with NGOs and initiate a local youth community to work and collaborate with others to bridge the gap of rural and urban.

Naw Pue Pue Mhote, also known as Tee Tar, is a Karen who works for the Burma Medical Association, a health group that serves ethnic communities. She was born in a rural community with little access to healthcare, so she knew how difficult it was to seek help. After high school, she crossed to Thailand by boat to learn how to treat sick people and joined her current organization. There, she encountered many people in desperate need of health care and education—basic human rights that had been denied to them owing to long-term armed conflicts. Witnessing her community's resiliency has inspired her to give back in every way possible.

NOTES

Story of Amy

- 1 in 4 Singaporeans marry non-residents[1].
- In 2022, there were 4,102 new marriages between resident groom and non-resident bride in Singapore. In comparison, in the same year there were 1,740 new marriages between resident bride and non-resident groom. These figures are relatively steady in last decade[2].

---

[1] Min, A.H. (2021) 1 in 4 Singaporeans marrying non-residents, increasing proportion involves non-resident men, CNA. Available at: https://www.channelnewsasia.com/singapore/singapore-citizen-marry-foreign-spouse-non-resident-236371 (Accessed: 04 November 2023).

[2] Marital status, marriages and divorces - latest data (2023) Department of Statistics Singapore. Available at: https://www.singstat.gov.sg/find-data/search-by-theme/population/marital-status-marriages-and-divorces/latest-data (Accessed: 04 November 2023).

- The most common pass (visa) type for a migrant spouse in Singapore are[3]:
  - LTVP (Long-Term Visit Pass): "sponsored by citizen spouse; valid for three months to two years; renewable; can apply for Letter of Consent (LOC) to work; qualifies for limited types of public housing; no access to healthcare subsidies"
  - LTVP+ (Long-Term Visit Pass Plus): "sponsored by citizen spouse; valid for three years at first, and up to five years upon renewal; can apply for LOC to work; qualifies for limited types of public housing; qualifies for some in-patient healthcare subsidies"

  If they cannot get LTVP, a migrant spouse will be on an employment-based pass if eligible or a short-visit pass (SVP) that is renewable for up to 89 days. SVP does not allow its holder to work or qualify for any form of public subsidies. Between 2012 and 2016, 13,900 migrant spouses of Singaporean citizens were granted LTVP out of 16,600 applications.
- Eligibility for employment-based pass includes a minimum salary of SGD 5,000 (or SGD 5,500 for the financial sector) which should increase progressively with age from age 23[3].

---

[3] Association of Women for Action and Research (2020) Migrant Wives in Distress: Issues facing non-resident women married to Singaporean men. rep. Singapore: AWARE.

- A foreigner can apply to become a permanent resident (PR) in Singapore if they fulfill the following requirements (quoted directly from source)[4]:
    o Spouse of a Singapore citizen or Singapore PR
    o Unmarried child aged below 21 years old, born within the context of a legal marriage to, or have been legally adopted by, a Singapore citizen or PR
    o Aged parent of a Singapore citizen
    o Holder of an Employment Pass or S Pass
    o Student studying in Singapore
    o Foreign investor in Singapore
- The five most common issues reported by migrant wives in Singapore are about divorce, family violence, children's custody, uncertainty over the right to reside in Singapore, and housing[3].
- The highest levels of within-family conflict and the lowest monthly income per capita in Singapore are experienced by mix-nationality families with a foreign mother/wife and a citizen father/husband. Foreign wives on LTVP are especially disadvantaged socio-economically[5].

---

[4] Becoming a permanent resident, Immigration & Checkpoints Authority Singapore. Available at: https://www.ica.gov.sg/reside/PR/apply (Accessed: 04 November 2023).

[5] Tan, T. (2021) 'New study sheds light on cross-national families in S'pore', The Straits Times, 18 January. Available at https://fass.nus.edu.sg/cfpr/wp-content/uploads/sites/17/2021/01/18Jan2021_ST.pdf

Story of Habib

- The Rohingya are a Muslim ethnic minority group who have lived for centuries in predominantly Buddhist Myanmar - formerly known as Burma. Despite living in Myanmar for many generations, the Rohingya are not recognized as an official ethnic group and have been denied citizenship since 1982, making them the world's largest stateless population[6].
- The Rohingya have suffered decades of violence, discrimination and persecution in Myanmar[6].
- In August 2017, armed attacks, massive scale violence, and serious human rights violations forced thousands of Rohingya to flee their homes in Myanmar's Rakhine State. Many walked for days through jungles and undertook dangerous sea journeys across the Bay of Bengal to reach safety in Bangladesh. Now, more than 960,000 people have found safety in Bangladesh with a majority living in the Cox Bazar's region - home to the world's largest refugee camp[6].
- The Rohingya fleeing attacks and violence in the 2017 exodus joined around 300,000 people already in Bangladesh from previous waves of

---

[6] Rohingya Rufugee Crisis Explained, dated 23 August 2023. Available at https://www.unrefugees.org/news/rohingya-refugee-crisis-explained/#RohingyainBangladesh (Accessed: 27 Dec 2023)

displacement, effectively forming the world's largest refugee camp[7].

- The monsoon season in Bangladesh runs from June to October each year and brings heavy rainfall and strong wind, increasing the risk of floods and landslides. Hundreds of thousands of Rohingya have found refuge in flimsy shelters made of bamboo and tarp which have been built in areas prone to landslides, which may not stand torrential rains and heavy winds. The rainy season also exacerbates the risk of disease - such as hepatitis, malaria, dengue and chikungunya - in crowded camps that don't have proper water and sanitation facilities, putting children and the elderly at particular risk[8].

- Starting from the 1st June 2023, the funding shortages forced the World Food Programme (WFP) to reduce food assistance for the Rohingya refugees in Cox's Bazar from USD 10 to USD 8 per month, just three months since the first round of cut. This reduction in ration will push the current food assistance provided to the Rohingyas fall far below the recognized global humanitarian standard of 2,100 kcal, entailing a significant drop in refugees' food intake. Even before the first round of food ration cut in March 2023, with WFP's food assistance,

---

[7] Rohingya Crisis, UNICEF. Available at https://www.unicef.org/emergencies/rohingya-crisis (Accessed: 27 Dec 2023)

four in 10 families were not consuming enough food and 12 percent of children were acutely malnourished[8].
- Simultaneously, Water, Sanitation and Hygiene (WASH) sector has to decrease the number of bathing soaps for Rohingya refugees to one per person per month from 1 June 2023 as well[8].
- Cuts in essential humanitarian assistance have severe impacts on the refugees and the host community, which lead potentially to criminal activities, such as theft and robbery, increased domestic violence, gender-based violence, and neglect towards persons with disabilities and older individuals in the community. These cuts may also result in further social tension or conflict among communities as resources will be limited or overstretched[8].

---

[8] Decreasing humanitarian assistance threatens the life of 1 million Rohingya refugees in Bangladesh: food ration and soap cuts, Reliefweb. Available at https://reliefweb.int/report/bangladesh/decreasing-humanitarian-assistance-threatens-life-1-million-rohingya-refugees-bangladesh-food-ration-and-soap-cuts (Accessed: 27 Dec 2023)

Story of Mok

- Singapore is currently one of the most rapidly aging country in Asia. 16.6% of Singaporean residents are of age 65 or above[9].
- The number of elderly Singaporean residents who live alone increased 36% from 2018 to 2022. In 2022, there are 78,000 elderly who live alone. This number is expected to keep increasing in the future[10].
- Some elderly Singaporean residents are more at risk to live alone than others. Elderly women living alone has increased by 40% in the last 1.5 decades. Living alone is also correlated with having no living children, widowhood or never being married, low socioeconomic status, and the wish to be independent[11].
- The prevalence of depressive symptoms is higher amongst elderly Singaporean residents who live

---

[9] Statista Research Department. (2023) Singapore: Elderly share of resident population 2022, Statista. Available at: https://www.statista.com/statistics/1112943/singapore-elderly-share-of-resident-population/ (Accessed: 04 November 2023).

[10] Ministry of Health Singapore (2023) Seniors Staying Alone, Ministry of Health. Available at: https://www.moh.gov.sg/news-highlights/details/seniors-staying-alone (Accessed: 04 November 2023).

[11] Linton, E., Gubhaju, B. and Chan, A. (2018) Research brief series : 4 - Home Alone: Older Adults in Singapore, Centre for Ageing Research and Education. Available at: https://www.duke-nus.edu.sg/docs/librariesprovider3/research-policy-brief-docs/home-alone-older-adults-in-singapore.pdf

alone compared to those who live with children. However, this also depends on the strength of social network outside of the home. There is association between less depressive symptoms and stronger social network[11].
- Elderly Singaporean residents see successful ageing as "being happy, healthy, physically active, financially independent, and having close friendships"[12].

Story of Zhao

- 45% of middle-aged and elderly people in China live with hearing loss. The risk factors related to hearing loss amongst these age groups in China include advanced age itself, exposure to noise, gender (the prevalence in males is slightly higher than females), ear and metabolic diseases, and use of medication with side effects affecting hearing[13].

---

[12] Mathews, M. and Straughan, P.T. (2014) Results from the perception and attitudes towards ageing and seniors survey (2013/2014). Singapore Management University. Available at: https://ink.library.smu.edu.sg/soss_research/2220/

[13] Gong, R. *et al.* (2018) 'Hearing loss prevalence and risk factors among older adults in China', *International Journal of Audiology*, 57(5), pp. 354–359. doi:10.1080/14992027.2017.1423404.

- Amongst Chinese working age adults (25-59), being unemployed or a blue-collar worker and low education are associated with hearing loss[14].
- Of all human hearing loss cases, approximately 90% are of a type called sensorineural hearing loss where there are damages on the nerve system or structure needed for hearing in either the ears or the brain. Of these cases in China, genetic factors have around 60% contribution to the condition but 40% is contributed by environmental or other unknown factors[15,16].
- People with hearing loss in China experience higher unemployment rate, lower educational status, and tend to come from low-income families[17].
- A 2022 study in China found that people with hearing loss aged 45+ who were given

---

[14] He, P. *et al.* (2018) 'Association of Socioeconomic Status with hearing loss in Chinese working-aged adults: A population-based study', *PLOS ONE*, 13(3). doi:10.1371/journal.pone.0195227.

[15] Tanna, R.J., Lin, J.W. and Jesus, O.D. (2023) *Sensorineural hearing loss*, *National Library of Medicine*. Available at: https://www.ncbi.nlm.nih.gov/books/NBK565860/ (Accessed: 04 November 2023).

[16] Yuan, Y. *et al.* (2019) 'Comprehensive genetic testing of Chinese SNHL patients and variants interpretation using ACMG guidelines and ethnically matched normal controls', *European Journal of Human Genetics*, 28(2), pp. 231–243. doi:10.1038/s41431-019-0510-6.

[17] Deaf People and Human Rights, by Ms Hilde Haualand and Mr Colin Allen for the World Federation of the Deaf and the Swedish National Association of the Deaf, 2009

hearing aids experienced reduced expenses in self-medication healthcare compared to those who weren't - potentially due to their improved ability to understand and follow recommended treatment from the formal health system. However, this difference was only observed amongst those with better social network and those from middle-age group (45-65)[18].

- (Hearing) children of deaf adults (CODA) in China also have unique lived experiences. The experience of "inversion of the parent-child dynamic" and extended stigma can contribute to some of them feeling like they are "marginal figures caught between two separate worlds". However, their existence also contribute to them being "a bridge that brings these worlds together", for example through their ability to act as sign-language interpreters[19].

---

[18] Ye, X. *et al.* (2023) 'Impacts of the hearing aid intervention on healthcare utilization and costs among middle-aged and older adults: Results from a randomized controlled trial in rural China', *The Lancet Regional Health - Western Pacific*, 31, p. 100594. doi:10.1016/j.lanwpc.2022.100594.

[19] Zuan, Z. (2022) *China's CODA share their stories*, *#SixthTone*. Available at: https://www.sixthtone.com/news/1010204 (Accessed: 04 November 2023)

Story of Arun

- The term 'dementia' is generally used for a decline in mental ability that is severe enough to disturb daily life, while 'Alzheimer's' refers specifically to a type of degenerative disease caused by complex brain changes due to cellular damage. 60-80% of dementia cases are due to Alzheimer's[20].
- It is estimated that there are currently about 600,000 people with dementia in Thailand, a number which can reach 1 million by 2030[21].
- Old age is one of the main risk factors for Alzheimer's. However, this condition does not have a single cause. Various factors can contribute to its development, such as genetics, lifestyle, environment, social, metabolic

---

[20] Alzheimer's Association (no date) Dementia vs. Alzheimer's disease: What is the difference?, Alzheimer's Disease and Dementia. Available at: https://www.alz.org/alzheimers-dementia/difference-between-dementia-and-alzheimer-s (Accessed: 04 November 2023).

[21] Alzheimer's Disease International and Alzheimer's Australia (2014) Dementia in the Asia Pacific Region. rep. London: Alzheimer's Disease International. Available at: https://www.alzint.org/u/Dementia-Asia-Pacific-2014.pdf

- diseases, history of head injury, or other brain diseases[22,23,24].
- Amongst people with Alzheimer's, there are more women than men. However, it does not always mean women are inherently more at risk for Alzheimer's. This might be due to various reasons, such as women generally living longer than men, biological sex differences, risk factors experienced by or affecting men and women differently across the lifespan, unequal gender norms leading to less opportunities for lifelong mental stimulation, and others[25].
- In the last 1.5 decades, there are increasing levels and trends of household needs for caregivers for older people in Thailand. The lower-income

---

[22] Povova, J. et al. (2012) 'Epidemiological of and risk factors for alzheimer's disease: A Review', Biomedical Papers, 156(2), pp. 108–114. doi:10.5507/bp.2012.055.

[23] Mielke, M.M. et al. (2022) 'Traumatic brain injury and risk of alzheimer's disease and related dementias in the population', Journal of Alzheimer's Disease, 88(3), pp. 1049–1059. doi:10.3233/jad-220159.

[24] Xu, W. et al. (2015) 'Meta-analysis of modifiable risk factors for alzheimer's disease', Journal of Neurology, Neurosurgery & Psychiatry [Preprint]. doi:10.1136/jnnp-2015-310548.

[25] Mielke, M.M. (2018) Sex and gender differences in Alzheimer's disease dementia, The Psychiatric Times. Available at: https://www.ncbi.nlm.nih.gov/pmc/articles/PMC6390276/ (Accessed: 04 November 2023).

households and those in worse-off areas are more prone to have this need unmet[26].
- Informal caregivers are the main human resource providing dementia care in Thailand's rural area. Half of them are the adult children of the person with dementia, and most of them also had their own children. This multigenerational household means the caregivers could be trapped between providing the care for the elderly person with dementia and care for their own family. This situation can lead to financial, legal, and management issues, and also affect their physical and mental wellbeing[27].
- Thai's sandwich generation provide parental care mainly due to the value of gratitude[28].
- In Thailand, direct medical costs including for medications is the highest cost driver for Alzheimer's care. Alzheimer's medications in Thailand can only be prescribed in tertiary

---

[26] Phetsitong, R. and Vapattanawong, P. (2022) 'Household need and unmet need for caregivers of older persons in Thailand', Journal of Aging & Social Policy, 35(6), pp. 824–841. doi:10.1080/08959420.2022.2132081.

[27] Chuakhamfoo, N.N. et al. (2020) 'Health and long-term care of the elderly with dementia in rural Thailand: A cross-sectional survey through their caregivers', BMJ Open, 10(3). doi:10.1136/bmjopen-2019-032637.

[28] Vejbhumi, O. (2009) Parental caregiving among the sandwich generation in Bangkok metropolitan area. dissertation. National Institute of Development Administration. Available at: https://repository.nida.ac.th/items/3b14b066-a7fc-42c8-a485-d523e9c07d04

hospitals where Alzheimer's specialists are available[29].
- The second highest cost for Alzheimer's care in Thailand is indirect costs. This reflects that Alzheimer's generally contributes to a great economic burden for informal caregivers by incurring opportunity costs from lost of time. Additionally, the deterioration of physical and psychological wellbeing experienced by these caregivers are also higher compared to their non-caregiver peers[30].

Story of Yap

- The lifetime prevalence of mental health disorders in Singapore is 13.9%[31].
- During the COVID-19 pandemic, a survey amongst 21-49 years old individuals in Singapore showed prevalence rates of 8.7%,

---

[29] Kongpakwattana, K. et al. (2018) 'Compliance and persistence with alzheimer's disease treatment: A retrospective analysis of Multiregional Hospital databases in Thailand', Journal of Medical Economics, 22(1), pp. 26–34. doi:10.1080/13696998.2018.1534739.

[30] Kongpakwattana, K. et al. (2019) 'A real-world evidence analysis of associations among costs, quality of life, and disease-severity indicators of alzheimer's disease in Thailand', Value in Health, 22(10), pp. 1137–1145. doi:10.1016/j.jval.2019.04.1937.

[31] Mental Health in Singapore – statistics and facts. Available at https://www.statista.com/topics/10594/mental-health-in-singapore/#topicOverview

9.4%, and 9.3% for clinical depression, clinical anxiety, and mild to severe stress respectively[32].
- Cross-national families with a foreign-born mother/wife and a citizen father/husband in Singapore experience the highest levels of conflict within the family and the lowest monthly per capita income[5].
- In Singapore, there is still significant public stigma toward those with mental illness[33].
- Collectivist values, as well as the perceived "loss of face" if a person/family member is diagnosed with mental illness and the resultant loss of social capital, are concepts that are still present in several Asian cultures[34,35].
- Entwined with Asian cultural factors is the importance given to the concept of meritocracy in Singapore, which can lead to avoidance of getting a diagnosis and asccessing treatment

---

[32] COVID-19 Mental Wellness Taskforce Report, by MOH and IMH. Available https://www.moh.gov.sg/docs/librariesprovider5/covid-19-report/comwt-report.pdf

[33] Tan, G.T.H., Shahwan, S., Goh, C.M.J. *et al.* Mental illness stigma's reasons and determinants (MISReaD) among Singapore's lay public – a qualitative inquiry. *BMC Psychiatry* **20**, 422 (2020). https://doi.org/10.1186/s12888-020-02823-6

[34] Yang LH, Kleinman A. 'Face' and the embodiment of stigma in China: the cases of schizophrenia and AIDS. *Soc Sci Med.* 2008;67(3):398-408. doi:10.1016/j.socscimed.2008.03.011

[35] Papadopoulos C, Foster J, Caldwell K. 'Individualism-collectivism' as an explanatory device for mental illness stigma. *Community Ment Health J.* 2013;49(3):270-280. doi:10.1007/s10597-012-9534-x

due to not wanting to belong to the "Other" negatively stereotyped group or fear of losing social capital or future opportunities[34].

- In Singapore, home ownership is among the highest in the world. Citizens who have no other housing options are offered heavily subsidised rental housing. Residents staying in such rental housings are characterised by low socioeconomic status. Staying in public rental housing was found to be associated with poorer health status and outcomes in Singapore[36].

Story of Afina

- Epilepsy is the most common and one of the oldest human neurological conditions that can affect people of all ages. There are estimated 50 million people around the world who live with epilepsy[37].
- A generalized atonic seizure, one of the types of seizures in epilepsy, is "an epileptic drop attack, with sudden loss of muscle tone and strength

---

[36] Chan CQH, Lee KH, Low LL. A systematic review of health status, health seeking behaviour and healthcare utilisation of low socioeconomic status populations in urban Singapore. *Int J Equity Health*. 2018;17(1):39. Published 2018 Apr 2. doi:10.1186/s12939-018-0751-y/

[37] Banerjee, P.N., Filippi, D. and Allen Hauser, W. (2009) 'The descriptive epidemiology of epilepsy—a review', Epilepsy Research, 85(1), pp. 31–45. doi:10.1016/j.eplepsyres.2009.03.003.

and a fall to the ground or a slump in a chair". Its duration is usually only seconds[38].

- Commonly reported triggers for epileptic seizures include missing medication, sleep deprivation, emotional stress, and fatigue[39].
- Epilepsy is a severe and disabling condition that can - most of the time - be fully managed, but it is often associated with stigma, prejudice, and discrimination[40].
- People with epilepsy (and other chronic conditions) can be more at risk for discrimination and abuse, including sexual abuse[41].
- Stevens-Johnson syndrome (SJS) is "an acute and and potentially fatal skin reactions involving loss of skin and, in some cases, mucosal membranes [such as those inside the mouth and genitalia] accompanied by systemic symptoms".

---

[38] Fisher, R.S. (2017) 'The new classification of seizures by the International League Against Epilepsy 2017', Current Neurology and Neuroscience Reports, 17(6). doi:10.1007/s11910-017-0758-6.

[39] Nakken, K.O. et al. (2005) 'Which seizure-precipitating factors do patients with epilepsy most frequently report?', Epilepsy & Behavior, 6(1), pp. 85–89. doi:10.1016/j.yebeh.2004.11.003.

[40] Braga, P. et al. (2020) 'How to understand and address the cultural aspects and consequences of diagnosis of epilepsy, including stigma', Epileptic Disorders, 22(5), pp. 531–547. doi:10.1684/epd.2020.1201.

[41] Nimmo-Smith, V. et al. (2016) 'Discrimination, domestic violence, abuse, and other adverse life events in people with epilepsy: Population-based study to assess the burden of these events and their contribution to psychopathology', Epilepsia, 57(11), pp. 1870–1878. doi:10.1111/epi.13561.

Medications are the cause in more than 80% of cases. Medications that are correlated with the risk for SJS include anticonvulsants (such as antiepileptic medications), antibiotics, analgesics (pain medication), and antipyretics (medication for fever)[42].

Story of Rosa

- Schizophrenia is defined as "a mental disorder characterized by disruptions in thought processes, perceptions, emotional responsiveness, and social interactions". It is generally persistent and can be severe and disabling[43].
- In 2018, 7 in every 1,000 households in Indonesia has a member living with schizophrenia. This translates to approximately 470,000 individuals[44].
- Males with schizophrenia are generally found to have more severe clinical symptoms than

---

[42] Oakley, A.M. and Krishnamurthy, K. (2023) Stevens-Johnson Syndrome, National Library of Medicine. Available at: https://www.ncbi.nlm.nih.gov/books/NBK459323/ (Accessed: 04 November 2023).

[43] U.S. Department of Health and Human Services. (n.d.). *Schizophrenia*. National Institute of Mental Health. https://www.nimh.nih.gov/health/statistics/schizophrenia

[44] Badan Penelitian dan Pengembangan Kesehatan RI, 2018. Laporan Nasional Riskesdas 2018. Lembaga Penerbit Badan Penelitian dan Pengembangan Kesehatan, Jakarta.

females. However, there are still many complex gender-related differences (or lack thereof) that need further research[45].

- Stigma is an important challenge faced by people living with mental illness in Indonesia. The challenges introduced by stigmatization include challenges to active and equal participate in society, access to social services including healthcare, and the general ability to experience health and wellbeing[46]. Stigma also leads to experience of isolation, marginalization, rejection, discrimination, and even human rights violation[47].
- Stigma towards people living with mental illness like schizophrenia can have various different forms, such as but are not limited to personal (internalized) stigma, family stigma, public/

---

[45] Giordano, G. M., Bucci, P., Mucci, A., Pezzella, P., & Galderisi, S. (2021). Gender differences in clinical and psychosocial features among persons with schizophrenia: A mini review. *Frontiers in Psychiatry*, 12. https://doi.org/10.3389/fpsyt.2021.789179

[46] Rai, S.S. et al. (2020) 'Qualitative exploration of experiences and consequences of health-related stigma among Indonesians with HIV, leprosy, schizophrenia and diabetes', Kesmas: National Public Health Journal, 15(1). doi:10.21109/kesmas.v15i1.3306.

[47] Subu, M.A. *et al.* (2021) 'Types of stigma experienced by patients with mental illness and mental health nurses in Indonesia: A qualitative content analysis', *International Journal of Mental Health Systems*, 15(1). doi:10.1186/s13033-021-00502-x.

social stigma, and employment stigma[3]. This also includes stigma from healthcare providers[48].

- Amongst Indonesians, higher level of stigmatization towards people with mental illness is correlated with less knowledge or awareness about mental health and less experience or contact with mental illness. Interestingly higher level of education is not correlated with less stigmatization[49].
- The earliest version of the Indonesian Health Card introduced in 1999, is a government program aimed at providing access to healthcare services for the poor and vulnerable populations across the country. The card functions as a form of health insurance, covering various medical expenses such as consultations, examinations, medications, and hospitalization[50].
- The beneficiaries of the Indonesian Health Card are typically identified based on socioeconomic criteria, targeting those who are considered

---

[48] Abidin, S. and Irwanto, I. (2021) 'Stigma towards people with schizophrenia among the Health Study Students: Faculty of Medicine, Faculty of Psychology, and Department of Counseling in Jakarta', *IJDS: Indonesian Journal of Disability Studies*, 8(02), pp. 347–359. doi:10.21776/ub.ijds.2021.008.02.04.

[49] Hartini, N. *et al.* (2018) 'Stigma toward people with mental health problems in Indonesia', *Psychology Research and Behavior Management*, Volume 11, pp. 535–541. doi:10.2147/prbm.s175251.

[50] Sparrow R. Targeting the poor in times of crisis: the Indonesian health card. Health Policy Plan. 2008 May;23(3):188-99. doi: 10.1093/heapol/czn003. Epub 2008 Mar 11. PMID: 18334517.

financially disadvantaged. Once enrolled, cardholders can access healthcare services at registered healthcare facilities, including public hospitals and clinics, without having to pay out-of-pocket expenses covered by the program.
- Mental health services in Indonesia still experience accessibility challenges due to various reasons - amongst all the low number and unequal spread of mental health professionals, stigma, mental health literacy amongst both the public and professionals, low public funding, and lack of interprofessional collaboration[51].
- People living with schizophrenia in Indonesia still face barriers to healthcare services. In 2018, although 84.9% of Indonesians with schizophrenia received some kind of treatment, more than half are not on continuous treatment[43]. Despite being banned by a new mental health law passed in 2014, the practice of inhumane confinement or 'pasung' still exists[52].
- While cultural and religious values do influence perception of mental illness and its 'solutions' amongst Indonesians - including by exacerbating stigma and increasing people's

---

[51] Putri, A.K. *et al.* (2021) 'Exploring the perceived challenges and support needs of Indonesian mental health stakeholders: A qualitative study', *International Journal of Mental Health Systems*, 15(1). doi:10.1186/s13033-021-00504-9.

[52] *Indonesia: Pasung Sudah Berkurang, Namun Tetap Ada.* (2023). Human Rights Watch. Available at: https://www.hrw.org/id/news/2018/10/02/322930 (Accessed: 04 November 2023).

hesitance to access services in the formal healthcare system - cultural acceptability and appropriateness of mental health services remain a work-in-progress to close the gap between people living with mental illness and the care they need, for which some efforts are currently ongoing[53,54].

---

[53] Bouman, T.K., Lommen, M.J.J. and Setiyawati, D. (2022) 'The acceptability of cognitive behaviour therapy in Indonesian Community Health Care', *The Cognitive Behaviour Therapist*, 15. doi:10.1017/s1754470x22000228.

[54] Renwick, L. *et al.* (2023) 'Culturally adapted family intervention for people with schizophrenia in Indonesia (fusion): A development and feasibility study protocol', *Pilot and Feasibility Studies*, 9(1). doi:10.1186/s40814-023-01280-8.

ACKNOWLEDGEMENTS

Our heartfelt thanks to the team at the Equity Initiative Programme for encouraging, guiding, mentoring and supporting us to put together this book sharing stories of persons living in our region, living in poor health and shine a light on their lived experiences and vulnerabilities. We are proud to be Senior Fellows of the Equity Initiative Programme and the Atlantic Institute, which had been generously funded through the philanthropy of Chuck Feeney (read more about his life and vision in the book "Giving while Living").

We are grateful to Ms Anne Phelan for her guidance as an experienced editor to the Editorial team and her copyediting support, which gave us the confidence to move forward strongly with the initial versions of the manuscript.

A big thank you to the writers, story-owners and illustrators – without them this book would not be possible.

Finally we are eternally grateful to our families for their support, patience and encouragement throughout our work on this book.

Milton Keynes UK
Ingram Content Group UK Ltd.
UKHW031632201124
451457UK00005B/18

9 781543 782509